Endoscopic Management of Gastrointestinal Bleeding

Editor

IAN M. GRALNEK

GASTROINTESTINAL ENDOSCOPY CLINICS OF NORTH AMERICA

www.giendo.theclinics.com

Consulting Editor
CHARLES J. LIGHTDALE

July 2018 • Volume 28 • Number 3

ELSEVIER

1600 John F. Kennedy Boulevard • Suite 1800 • Philadelphia, Pennsylvania, 19103-2899

http://www.theclinics.com

GASTROINTESTINAL ENDOSCOPY CLINICS OF NORTH AMERICA Volume 28, Number 3
July 2018 ISSN 1052-5157, ISBN-13: 978-0-323-61064-3

Editor: Kerry Holland
Developmental Editor: Donald Mumford

Gastrointestinal Endoscopy Clinics of North America (ISSN 1052-5157) is published quarterly by Elsevier Inc., 360 Park Avenue South, New York, NY 10010-1710. Months of issue are January, April, July, and October. Business and Editorial Offices: 1600 John F. Kennedy Blvd., Suite 1800, Philadelphia, PA, 19103-2899. Periodicals postage paid at New York, NY and additional mailing offices. Subscription prices are $349.00 per year for US individuals, $593.00 per year for US institutions, $100.00 per year for US students and residents, $385.00 per year for Canadian individuals, $702.00 per year for Canadian institutions, $474.00 per year for international individuals, $702.00 per year for international institutions, and $245.00 per year for Canadian and foreign students/residents. To receive student/resident rate, orders must be accompanied by name of affiliated institution, date of term, and the *signature* of program/residency coordinator on institution letterhead. Orders will be billed at individual rate until proof of status is received. Foreign air speed delivery is included in all *Clinics* subscription prices. All prices are subject to change without notice. **POSTMASTER:** Send address change to *Gastrointestinal Endoscopy Clinics of North America*, Elsevier Health Sciences Division, Subscription Customer Service, 3251 Riverport Lane, Maryland Heights, MO 63043. **Customer Service: 1-800-654-2452 (US). From outside the United States, call 1-314-447-8871. Fax: 1-314-447-8029. E-mail: JournalsCustomerService-usa@elsevier.com (for print support) or JournalsOnlineSupport-usa@elsevier.com (for online support).**

Reprints. For copies of 100 or more, of articles in this publication, please contact the Commercial Reprints Department, Elsevier Inc., 360 Park Avenue South, New York, NY 10010-1710. Tel. 212-633-3874; Fax: 212-633-3820; E-mail: reprints@elsevier.com.

Gastrointestinal Endoscopy Clinics of North America is covered in *Excerpta Medica, MEDLINE/PubMed (Index Medicus), and MEDLINE/MEDLARS.*

Contributors

CONSULTING EDITOR

CHARLES J. LIGHTDALE, MD
Professor of Medicine, Division of Digestive and Liver Diseases, Columbia University
Medical Center, New York, New York, USA

EDITOR

IAN M. GRALNEK, MD, MSHS, FASGE
Chairman, Ellen and Pinchas Mamber Institute of Gastroenterology, Hepatology and
Nutrition, Emek Medical Center, Afula, Israel

AUTHORS

MAJID A. ALMADI, MBBS, FRCPC, MSc (Clinical Epidemiology)
Division of Gastroenterology, King Khalid University Hospital, King Saud University,
Riyadh, Saudi Arabia; Division of Gastroenterology, McGill University Health Center,
Montreal General Hospital, McGill University, Montreal, Quebec, Canada

ALAN N. BARKUN, MD, CM, FRCPC, MSc (Clinical Epidemiology)
Divisions of Gastroenterology and Clinical Epidemiology, McGill University Health Center,
Montreal General Hospital, McGill University, Montreal, Quebec, Canada

KENDALL R. BECK, MD
Assistant Professor, Department of Medicine, Division of Gastroenterology, University of
California, San Francisco, San Francisco, California, USA

ALLAN I. BLOOM, MD, FSIR
Director of Vascular and Interventional Radiology, Department of Radiology, Hadassah
University Medical Center, Ein Karem, Jerusalem, Israel

JENNIFER X. CAI, MD, MPH
Division of Gastroenterology, Hepatology and Endoscopy, Brigham and Women's
Hospital, Harvard Medical School, Boston, Massachusetts, USA

FRANCIS K.L. CHAN, MD
Professor, Department of Medicine and Therapeutics, Prince of Wales Hospital, Shatin,
Hong Kong

MICHAEL A. CHANG, MD
Assistant Clinical Professor of Medicine, Division of Gastroenterology, University of
California, San Diego, California, USA

KEVIN A. GHASSEMI, MD
Vatche and Tamar Manoukian Division of Digestive Diseases, David Geffen School of Medicine at UCLA, CURE: Digestive Diseases Research Center, Los Angeles, California, USA

DAVID A. GREENWALD, MD
Director of Clinical Gastroenterology and Endoscopy, Division of Gastroenterology, Professor of Medicine, Icahn School of Medicine at Mount Sinai, Mount Sinai Hospital, New York, New York, USA

SHIVANI GUPTA, MD
Division of Gastroenterology, Icahn School of Medicine at Mount Sinai, Mount Sinai Hospital, New York, New York, USA

HAZEM HAMMAD, MD
Gastroenterology Fellow, Division of Gastroenterology, University of Colorado Anschutz Medical Center, Denver, Colorado, USA

NAOKI ISHII, MD
Head, Division of Gastroenterology, Koga Hospital, Ibaraki, Japan

DENNIS M. JENSEN, MD
Vatche and Tamar Manoukian Division of Digestive Diseases, David Geffen School of Medicine at UCLA, CURE: Digestive Diseases Research Center, Department of Medicine, VA West Los Angeles Medical Center, Los Angeles, California, USA

TONYA KALTENBACH, MD, MS
Associate Professor, Clinical Medicine, University of California, San Francisco, Staff Physician, San Francisco VA Medical Center, San Francisco, California, USA

JENNIFER M. KOLB, MD
Gastroenterology Fellow, Division of Gastroenterology, University of Colorado Anschutz Medical Center, Denver, Colorado, USA

MOE H. KYAW, MBBS, MSc
Research Assistant Professor, Department of Medicine and Therapeutics, Prince of Wales Hospital, The Chinese University of Hong Kong, Shatin, Hong Kong

ALVARO MARTÍNEZ-ALCALÁ, MD
Department of Gastroenterology, Hospital Universitario Infanta Leonor, Madrid, Spain

KLAUS MÖNKEMÜLLER, MD, PhD, FASGE
Professor of Medicine, Department of Visceral Surgery, Division of Endoscopy, Frankenwaldklinik, Kronach, Germany

ZIV NEEMAN, MD
Chairman, Medical Imaging Institute, Haemek Medical Center, Afula, Israel

DAN E. ORRON, MD
Director of Vascular and Interventional Radiology, Department of Radiology, Carmel Medical Center, Haifa, Israel

JOHN R. SALTZMAN, MD, FACP, FACG, FASGE, AGAF
Division of Gastroenterology, Hepatology and Endoscopy, Director of Endoscopy, Brigham and Women's Hospital, Professor of Medicine, Harvard Medical School, Boston, Massachusetts, USA

THOMAS J. SAVIDES, MD
Professor of Medicine, Division of Gastroenterology, University of California, San Diego, California, USA

AMANDEEP K. SHERGILL, MD
Associate Professor, Department of Medicine, University of California, San Francisco, Department of Medicine, San Francisco VA Medical Center, San Francisco, California, USA

ROY SOETIKNO, MD, MS, MSM
Advanced GI Endoscopy, Mountain View, California, USA; Department of Gastroenterology, University of Indonesia, Jakarta, Indonesia

ADRIAN STANLEY, MD, FRCP
Consultant Gastroenterologist, Gastrointestinal Unit, Glasgow Royal Infirmary, Glasgow, United Kingdom

DEBBIE TROLAND, MB ChB, MRCP
Gastroenterology Specialist Trainee, Gastrointestinal Unit, Glasgow Royal Infirmary, Glasgow, United Kingdom

Contents

Inhospital mortality from nonvariceal upper gastrointestinal bleeding has improved with advances in medical and endoscopy therapy. Initial management includes resuscitation, hemodynamic monitoring, proton pump inhibitor therapy, and restrictive blood transfusion. Risk stratification scores help triage bleeding severity and provide prognosis. Upper endoscopy is recommended within 24 hours of presentation; select patients at lowest risk may be effectively treated as outpatients. Emergent endoscopy within 12 hours does not improve clinical outcomes, including mortality, rebleeding, or need for surgery, despite an increased use of endoscopic treatment. There may be a benefit to emergent endoscopy in patients with evidence of active bleeding.

Peptic ulcer bleeding is common and associated with significant morbidity and mortality. The authors discuss the endoscopic assessment of peptic ulcers and the rationale for treatment. They also review the evidence for the available endoscopic therapies, both individually and in combination, to draw conclusions on the optimum endoscopic management of peptic ulcer bleeding.

Nonvariceal, nonulcer upper gastrointestinal hemorrhage (UGIH) is a less common cause for acute upper gastrointestinal bleeding. However, nonvariceal, nonulcer UGIH is an important entity to identify and treat appropriately to prevent bleeding-related morbidity and mortality. Over the past 40 years, there has been a revolution in gastrointestinal endoscopy and a similar revolution in the management of UGIH. This article discusses the endoscopic management of nonvariceal, nonulcer UGIH, with a focus on the newer diagnostic and treatment modalities currently available.

Despite major improvements in endoscopic devices and therapeutic endoscopy, rebleeding rates and mortality have remained the same for several decades. Therefore, much interest has been paid to emerging therapeutic devices, such as the over-the-scope clip and hemostatic sprays. Other emerging technologies, such as radiofrequency ablation, endoscopic suturing devices, and ultrasound-guided angiotherapy, are also being investigated to improve therapeutic outcomes in specific situations. This article details the technical aspects, clinical applications, outcomes, and potential limitations of these devices in the context of nonvariceal upper gastrointestinal hemorrhage.

This article examines the use of the Doppler endoscopic probe (DEP) for risk stratification and as a guide to definitive hemostasis of nonvariceal upper gastrointestinal bleeding and colonic diverticular hemorrhage. Studies report that lesions with high-risk stigmata of recent hemorrhage (SRH) have a higher rate of a positive DEP signal compared with those without such SRH. Lesions with a persistently positive DEP signal after endoscopic hemostasis have a higher 30-day rebleeding rate. Studies document arterial blood flow underneath stigmata of recent hemorrhage as a risk factor for rebleeding of focal nonvariceal gastrointestinal lesions. With DEP probe as a guide, rates of definitive endoscopic hemostasis and clinical outcomes are improved compared with standard visually guided treatment.

Nearly 50 years ago, catheter angiography was introduced as a means of both diagnosing and treating nonvariceal upper gastrointestinal bleeding. Technologic advances and innovations have resulted in the introduction of microcatheters that, using a coaxial technique, are capable of selecting third-order arterial branches and of delivering a wide array of embolic agents. This article reviews the imaging diagnosis of nonvariceal upper gastrointestinal bleeding, the techniques of diagnostic and therapeutic angiography, the angiographic appearance of the various causes of nonvariceal upper gastrointestinal bleeding, the rationale behind case-specific selection of embolic agents, as well as the anticipated outcome of transcatheter arterial embolization.

The incidence of antithrombotic-associated gastrointestinal (GI) bleeding is increasing owing to the growing advanced-age population. There is consensus on ceasing anticoagulant and antiplatelet agents during an acute GI bleeding episode, but clearer guidance is needed on resumption of these agents. This article reviews evidence for optimal management of antithrombotics in the setting of acute GI bleeding and highlights areas in which future studies are needed.

Section II – Acute Lower Gastrointestinal Hemorrhage

Majid A. Almadi and Alan N. Barkun

The approach to lower gastrointestinal bleeding (LGIB) has evolved over the last few years to incorporate a multidisciplinary management strategy. Although the causes of LGIB vary depending on the age and comorbid conditions of patients, the initial resuscitation and principles of optimizing patients' condition before endoscopic evaluation, when appropriate, are the cornerstones to clinical care. The role of risk stratification is to triage patients as well as to mobilize health care resources based on predicted outcomes. Individualized management according to patients' comorbid conditions has been a focus in most recent guidelines.

Kendall R. Beck and Amandeep K. Shergill

Lower gastrointestinal bleeding is bleeding from a colonic source. Rapid colon purge using 4 to 6 L of polyethylene glycol followed by early colonoscopy, within 24 hours of presentation, is recommended to optimize the detection and management of bleeding sources. Although the data are mixed, early colonoscopy seems to be associated with higher detection of bleeding lesions and therapeutic interventions. There is no clear benefit for early colonoscopy in terms of reduced duration of stay, rebleeding, transfusion requirement, or surgery compared with patients undergoing elective colonoscopy. Further studies are needed to determine the effect of early colonoscopy on clinically important outcomes.

Roy Soetikno, Naoki Ishii, Jennifer M. Kolb, Hazem Hammad, and Tonya Kaltenbach

Acute severe lower gastrointestinal bleeding (LGIB) can be treated by endoscopy safely and effectively. At present, the data on the efficacy of endoscopy in the treatment of patients with LGIB are still being collected. Thus, guidelines to manage patients with LGIB are still in development. Herein, based on the recent literature and their 20-year experience in their units in the United States and in Japan, the authors summarize the role of endoscopic hemostasis therapy in acute severe LGIB with a focus on how to perform the hemostasis techniques.

This article summarizes current knowledge regarding the incidence of and risk factors associated with recurrent lower gastrointestinal hemorrhage. The literature regarding medical, endoscopic, and surgical methods to prevent rebleeding from diverticulosis, angioectasia, and chronic hemorrhagic radiation proctopathy is reviewed. In addition, the evidence for endoscopic clipping as primary prophylaxis against postpolypectomy bleeding is explored.

GASTROINTESTINAL ENDOSCOPY CLINICS OF NORTH AMERICA

THE CLINICS ARE AVAILABLE ONLINE!
Access your subscription at:
www.theclinics.com

Foreword

Upper and Lower Gastrointestinal Bleeding: Everything You Need to Know

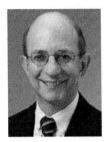

Charles J. Lightdale, MD
Consulting Editor

Hematemesis, melena, hematochezia, the presenting symptoms of acute gastrointestinal (GI) bleeding, are frightening to the patient and a call to action for gastrointestinal endoscopists. While the initial resuscitation of the patient with acute GI bleeding usually is accomplished by emergency medical specialists, it takes highly trained endoscopists to determine the location and cause of the bleeding source and in many instances to apply endoscopic therapy to stop the hemorrhage and prevent its recurrence.

This issue of *Gastrointestinal Endoscopy Clinics of North America* is devoted to the "Endoscopic Management of Gastrointestinal Bleeding," and the editor of the issue, Dr Ian M. Gralnek, is a world-renowned leader in gastroenterology with a research focus in both upper and lower gastrointestinal hemorrhage, and thus uniquely qualified to present this comprehensive review. He has gathered an international group of expert authors covering in detail the critical initial assessment of the patient with GI bleeding, standard endoscopic therapies and new treatment approaches, and the determination of when and how to apply colonoscopy and endoscopic hemostasis in lower GI bleeding. This is an issue packed with essential and cutting-edge information not to be missed by GI endoscopists from trainees to senior attending specialists. Read this issue and keep the articles accessible for reference on your computer and mobile device. You will be up-to-date, and you will sleep better on-call, knowing

Gastrointest Endoscopy Clin N Am 28 (2018) xiii–xiv
https://doi.org/10.1016/j.giec.2018.04.002
1052-5157/18/© 2018 Published by Elsevier Inc.

giendo.theclinics.com

that if the phone rings, you will be fully informed and ready to manage the patient with GI bleeding.

Charles J. Lightdale, MD
Department of Medicine
Columbia University Medical Center
161 Fort Washington Avenue
New York, NY 10032, USA

E-mail address:
CJL18@columbia.edu

Preface

Endoscopic Management of Gastrointestinal Bleeding

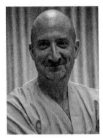

Ian M. Gralnek, MD, MSHS, FASGE
Editor

Acute gastrointestinal (GI) bleeding is one of the most common clinical problems encountered in gastroenterology and all too frequently rousts many a gastroenterologist from their slumber when on call. The most common type of acute GI bleeding is *upper* GI bleeding. However, recent data show that acute *lower* GI bleeding is not far behind in incidence, especially as the population ages and the use of antithrombotic medications increases. Thus, this issue of *Gastrointestinal Endoscopy Clinics of North America* is divided into two specific sections: Section I, which is a review of the management of acute nonvariceal upper GI bleeding (NVUGIB), and Section II, a review of the management of acute lower GI bleeding.

Acute NVUGIB may originate from the esophagus, stomach, or duodenum, essentially anywhere proximal to the ligament of Treitz. Drs Cai and Saltzman from the Brigham and Women's Hospital and Harvard Medical School in Boston, Massachusetts begin this issue with a review of patient presentation/initial assessment, risk stratification, and how to initially manage patients with acute NVUGIB. As we all know, endoscopic hemostasis is the standard of care for most of these patients. Moreover, peptic ulcer bleeding is the most common cause of NVUGIB; thus, Drs Troland and Stanley, from the Glasgow Royal Infirmary in Glasgow, Scotland provide an in-depth, evidence-based review of the endoscopic management of peptic ulcer bleeding. Drs Chang and Savides from the University of California at San Diego review the endoscopic management of all other causes of acute NVUGIB, such as Dieulafoy lesion, arteriovenous malformation, Mallory-Weiss tear, and malignant lesions. In addition, Drs Martínez-Alcalá and Mönkemüller, from Madrid, Spain and Kronbach, Germany, respectively, discuss emerging endoscopic hemostasis treatments, such as topical sprays, over-the-scope clipping devices, and more! In addition, there is a very interesting article from Drs Ghassemi and Jensen from the University of California at Los Angeles detailing the emerging provocative data on the role of Doppler ultrasound in guiding endoscopic hemostasis therapy. Although endoscopic

Gastrointest Endoscopy Clin N Am 28 (2018) xv–xvi
https://doi.org/10.1016/j.giec.2018.04.001
1052-5157/18/© 2018 Published by Elsevier Inc.

giendo.theclinics.com

hemostasis is highly effective, there are cases where bleeding is unable to be controlled or when significant rebleeding occurs that is not amenable to endoscopic therapy. Therefore, I have included an article that provides insight into the question, "what if endoscopic hemostasis fails?" submitted by our interventional radiology colleagues, Drs Orron, Bloom, and Neeman from Israel. This article details the role of radiologic evaluation and angiographic embolization in NVUGIH, which has now emerged as the oft-preferred salvage treatment strategy over surgical intervention. Last, Drs Kyaw and Chan, from the Prince of Wales Hospital and Chinese University of Hong Kong, focus on managing antithrombotic agents in the setting of acute GI bleeding.

In Section II of this issue, the focus is on the management of acute lower GI bleeding. We begin with a review of patient presentation, risk stratification, and initial management of patients presenting with acute lower GI bleeding by Drs Almadi and Barkun from King Khalid University Hospital, King Saud University, Riyadh, Saudi Arabia, and the McGill University Health Center, Montreal General Hospital, McGill University, Montréal, Canada. This is followed by a very nice article by Drs Beck and Shergill from the University of California at San Francisco discussing the role of colonoscopy in acute lower GI bleeding. Specifically, the role of colonoscopy in diagnosis, timing of colonocopy, and what appropriate bowel preparation to use in the acute lower GI bleeding patient. Then, Drs Soetikno, Kaltenbach, and colleagues provide important insight into the role of endoscopic hemostasis in lower GI bleeding and discuss the various hemostasis modalities we have at our disposal and what may work best in this specific patient population. Last, Drs Gupta and Greenwald from the Icahn School of Medicine at Mount Sinai in New York City review strategies for the prevention of recurrent lower GI bleeding.

I am sincerely grateful to all the authors who so willingly contributed to this issue. Of note, this is a true international effort since the distinguished authors of this issue come from North America, Europe, and Asia and graciously provide their clinical expertise on this very important topic. We have attempted to put together a comprehensive issue on "Endoscopic Management of Gastrointestinal Bleeding," and I hope that you will find this issue as informative and helpful in your practice as I have.

Enjoy!

Ian M. Gralnek, MD, MSHS, FASGE
Ellen and Pinchas Mamber Institute of
Gastroenterology, Hepatology and Nutrition
Emek Medical Center
Afula, Israel

E-mail address:
ian_gr@clalit.org.il

Initial Assessment, Risk Stratification, and Early Management of Acute Nonvariceal Upper Gastrointestinal Hemorrhage

Jennifer X. Cai, MD, MPH, John R. Saltzman, MD*

KEYWORDS

- Nonvariceal upper gastrointestinal bleeding • Upper endoscopy
- Proton-pump inhibitor • Risk stratification • Clinical management
- Nasogastric lavage • Video capsule endoscopy • Timing of endoscopy

KEY POINTS

- Initial management of nonvariceal upper gastrointestinal bleeding (UGIB) includes fluid resuscitation, hemodynamic monitoring, proton pump inhibitor therapy, and a restrictive blood transfusion strategy.
- Upper endoscopy is recommended in patients with nonvariceal UGIB within 24 hours of presentation; however, patients at lowest risk (ie, Glasgow-Blatchford score of 0–1) may be effectively treated as outpatients.
- Emergent endoscopy within 12 hours should be performed only after adequate resuscitation; however, it remains controversial. Emergent endoscopy has generally not been shown to significantly improve clinical outcomes, including mortality, rebleeding, or need for surgery, compared with endoscopy within 24 hours.

INTRODUCTION

Nonvariceal upper gastrointestinal bleeding (UGIB) is a common cause of hospitalization and accounts for more than 300,000 inpatient admissions in the United States annually.[1] For more than 50 years, the mortality from UGIB had been reported at 5% to 14%; however, recent evidence suggests that inhospital mortality has decreased to around 2%, likely due to advances in medical and endoscopic treatment.[1–4] The management of nonvariceal UGIB remains a significant and rising

---

Disclosure Statement: The authors have no financial relationships to disclose.

Division of Gastroenterology, Hepatology and Endoscopy, Brigham and Women's Hospital, Harvard Medical School, 75 Francis Street, Boston, MA 02115, USA

* Corresponding author.

E-mail address: jsaltzman@bwh.harvard.edu

Gastrointest Endoscopy Clin N Am 28 (2018) 261–275
https://doi.org/10.1016/j.giec.2018.02.001
1052-5157/18/© 2018 Elsevier Inc. All rights reserved.

economic burden; expenditures in the United States increased from $3.3 billion in 1989 to $7.6 billion in 2009.[2]

The initial management of patients with nonvariceal UGIB includes placement of 2 large-bore intravenous (IV) catheters, resuscitation, close hemodynamic monitoring, administration of proton-pump inhibitors (PPIs), and consideration of blood transfusion. Following adequate resuscitation, performing an upper endoscopy is typically the next step. Current guidelines recommend that endoscopy be performed within 24 hours of presentation; however, the most appropriate timing of endoscopy, particularly in higher risk patients, has been debated.[5–9] Risk stratification scores and other adjunctive techniques, including nasogastric (NG) lavage and video capsule endoscopy (VCE) have been used to triage the severity of bleeding as well as provide diagnostic and prognostic information for further management. This article reviews the existing literature on the initial assessment, risk stratification, and early management of nonvariceal UGIB.

RESUSCITATION AND MONITORING

Adequate resuscitation and stabilization is a critical first step in managing patients with UGIB. Venous access should be established immediately, with 2 large-caliber (18 gauge or larger) peripheral IV catheters to maximize flow rate, although a central venous catheter may be needed in patients who have difficult peripheral access. Fluids (ie, normal saline or lactated Ringer solution) should then be infused to restore a normal circulating blood volume. In patients with hemodynamic instability, such as those exhibiting shock or orthostatic hypotension, rapid IV fluid should be administered and vasopressor therapy should be considered. In addition, supplemental oxygen via nasal cannula is often given. Most patients who are hemodynamically stable following initial resuscitation may be admitted to a regular hospital ward; however, for patients who remain hemodynamically unstable, have respiratory compromise, with multiple comorbidities, and/or have active bleeding manifested by large-volume or ongoing hematemesis, admission to the intensive care unit (ICU) is recommended for closer monitoring.[10]

Prophylactic endotracheal intubation in select patients with nonvariceal UGIB has also been advocated to mitigate the risk of cardiopulmonary adverse events, such as aspiration pneumonia from massive hematemesis or volume overload following resuscitation. However, a recent study of 200 adults with hematemesis and/or melena with consequential hypovolemic shock revealed that overall cardiopulmonary unplanned event rates were significantly higher in subjects who were preemptively intubated compared with a propensity-matched cohort of subjects who were not intubated (20% vs 6%, $P = .008$).[11] The higher incidence of cardiopulmonary adverse events in the intubated group was largely driven by a higher percentage of intubated patients who developed pneumonia and shock (both 14%) as compared with nonintubated subjects (2% and 6%, respectively). These results suggest that prophylactic endotracheal intubation for a brisk UGIB in critically ill subjects, who are also those most often considered for prophylactic intubation, may in fact lead to an increased risk of the very cardiopulmonary events that physicians hope to avoid. The decision to perform prophylactic endotracheal intubation must be individualized, carefully weighing both the possible benefits and potential risks.

PROTON-PUMP INHIBITOR THERAPY

Nonvariceal UGIB is primarily caused by damage to the gastric mucosa as a result of mucosal impairment and the presence of gastric acid and pepsin.[12] PPIs irreversibly block the secretion of gastric acid by inhibiting hydrogen potassium adenosine tri-phosphatase, thus elevating the stomach pH to facilitate clot stabilization, resulting in improved outcomes such as rebleeding, length of hospitalization, number of blood transfusions, and need for surgery.[13–18] Most current guidelines recommend an 80 mg IV bolus followed by an 8 mg/h continuous infusion of PPI; however, recent evidence suggest that continuous infusions are not more effective than high-dose intermittent PPI therapy, even in patients with high-risk stigmata UGIB.[19,20] Sachar and colleagues[21] performed a meta-analysis of 13 randomized controlled trials of subjects with Forrest class Ia to IIb lesions, revealing that intermittent PPI therapy was not inferior to continuous infusion with regard to rebleeding at 3 and 7 days, urgent intervention, need for surgical or repeat endoscopic intervention, or mortality.

The varying cost of different doses and frequency of PPI therapy has also been a consideration in guiding clinical practice. Lu and colleagues[22] performed a budget impact analysis to determine costs per patient presenting with nonvariceal UGIB from the perspective of a US third-party payer. The overall cost per patient was $11,399 when continuous IV PPI was initiated before endoscopy. The incremental savings was $106 if only postendoscopic continuous IV dosing was used, $223 in savings if both preendoscopy and postendoscopy intermittent IV doses were used, and $191 in savings if only postendoscopic intermittent IV PPI was used. This analysis suggests that the incremental costs of different IV PPI regimens are modest compared with the total cost per patient and favoring a dosing strategy over another should not primarily rely on cost considerations.

The authors currently manage admitted patients with nonvariceal UGIB with an IV bolus of a PPI, followed by intermittent IV dosing for 72 hours in patients who undergo endoscopic therapy or with high-risk endoscopic findings. In patients with low-risk findings at endoscopy, we manage with oral PPIs.

BLOOD TRANSFUSION

Transfusion of packed red blood cells is a key element in the initial management of UGIB, serving to maintain tissue perfusion, increase oxygen delivery, and replace blood volume in the setting of ongoing losses. Patients with exsanguinating bleeding, hypovolemic shock, and other evidence of tissue hypoperfusion (eg, cardiac demand ischemia), or significant active bleeding will require blood transfusion regardless of hemoglobin level because hemoglobin values on presentation have not yet had time to equilibrate in cases of rapid bleeding. However, in stable patients with nonvariceal UGIB, the benefit of giving a blood transfusion to maximize oxygen-carrying capacity must be weighed against the risks of allergic reaction, transfusion-related acute lung injury, and volume overload.[10]

Guidelines have traditionally favored transfusing patients to a goal hemoglobin threshold of 9 to 10 g/dL; however, recent observational and retrospective studies have suggested that using a higher transfusion threshold actually resulted in worse outcomes.[23–25] Villanueva and colleagues[26] conducted a randomized controlled trial of 921 subjects with severe acute UGIB (including variceal bleeding). There were 225 subjects assigned to the restrictive strategy (transfuse for hemoglobin <7 g/dL) and 61 subjects assigned to the liberal strategy (transfuse for hemoglobin <9 g/dL) who did not receive blood transfusions. Mortality at 6 weeks, rebleeding, need for rescue therapy, and adverse event rates were all lower in the restrictive strategy group compared with the liberal transfusion group. It should be noted that the overall mortality benefit was driven by subjects with Child-Pugh class A and B cirrhosis, and that the subgroup of subjects with nonvariceal UGIB did not show a significant decrease in mortality with a restrictive transfusion strategy. Subjects with massive exsanguination, recent acute coronary syndrome, stroke, or transient ischemic attack were also excluded from the study.

Odutayo and colleagues[27] included 5 randomized controlled trials with 1965 subjects (including those with cirrhosis and ischemic heart disease) in a recent meta-analysis comparing restrictive and liberal transfusion strategies. Restrictive transfusion was associated with lower risk of all-cause mortality (relative risk [RR] 0.65, $P = .03$) and rebleeding (RR 0.58, $P = .004$). Based on these studies, it is reasonable to implement a restrictive policy of blood transfusion for subjects with nonvariceal UGIB with a threshold of hemoglobin level less than 7 g/dL, except in cases of massive active bleeding or cardiovascular comorbidities that may necessitate a more individualized strategy with higher transfusion thresholds of 9 to 10 g/dL.

RISK STRATIFICATION SCORES

Guidelines recommend the use of risk stratification scores to triage patients with UGIB to the appropriate level of care.[6,9,28] Several well-studied prognostic scales have been developed for this purpose, for both preendoscopic and postendoscopic use. The Glasgow-Blatchford score (GBS) and the AIMS65 score can both be calculated using only clinical data available on presentation, whereas the Rockall score requires endoscopic findings in addition to clinical data (**Table 1**).

The GBS was developed from a United Kingdom cohort of 1748 subjects with UGIB to predict their risk of requiring clinical intervention, including blood transfusion, endoscopy, or surgery.[29] Scores range from 0 to 23. A subsequent multicenter validation study by Stanley and colleagues[30] showed that patients with a GBS of 0 could be safely managed as outpatients without adverse events. Similarly, a meta-analysis of 25 studies found that a GBS of less than 2 was 98% sensitive for predicting no need for urgent evaluation of UGIB.[31] The 2015 European Society of Gastrointestinal Endoscopy guidelines recommend the use of the GBS for preendoscopy risk stratification and states that "outpatients determined to be at very low risk, based upon a GBS score of 0 - 1, do not require early endoscopy nor hospital admission."[9]

Compared with the GBS, the AIMS65 score has only 5 elements, each contributing 1 point to the total score, which can be easily calculated at the bedside and was predictive of inhospital death, length of stay (LOS), and cost in patients with acute UGIB.[32] The score was derived from 29,222 subjects and validated in 32,504 subjects with an area under the receiver operating characteristic (AUROC) curve of 0.77 (95% CI 0.75–0.79). Notably, the AIMS65 score predicts mortality, a clinically significant outcome, whereas the GBS predicts the need for clinical intervention, a surrogate outcome. Subjects with an AIMS65 score of 0 or 1 had a low rate of mortality (0.3% and 1.2%, respectively) compared with those with a score of 4 or 5 (22% and 32%, respectively). A prospective study of 298 subjects found that the AIMS65 score was superior to the GBS for predicting inhospital mortality and LOS in subjects with UGIB, yet similar for predicting 30-day mortality, inhospital rebleeding, and a composite outcome of inpatient mortality, transfusions, and need for intervention.[33]

The most widely used postendoscopic risk assessment tool is the Rockall score, which was developed from 4185 subjects using standardized questionnaires and found that age, shock, comorbidities, endoscopic diagnosis, and major stigmata of recent bleeding were independent predictors of mortality.[34] The Rockall score can be used as a full risk score or by only using the preendoscopy clinical parameters (see **Table 1**). Several studies have compared the Rockall score with the GBS and AIMS65 scores. In a cohort of 424 subjects, the AIMS65 score was found to be

Table 1
Components of the Glasgow-Blatchford, AIMS65, and Rockall scores

Risk Factor	Points
GBS	
BUN, mg/dL	
≥18.2–<22.4	2
≥22.4–<28.0	3
≥28.0–<70.0	4
≥70.0	6
Hemoglobin, men, g/dL	
≥12.0–<13.0	1
≥10.0–<12.0	3
<10.0	6
Hemoglobin, women, g/dL	
≥10.0–<12.0	1
<10.0	6
SBP, mm Hg	
100–109	1
90–99	2
<90	3
Other clinical parameters	
Heart rate ≥100 bpm	1
Melena	1
Syncope	2
Liver disease	2
CHF	2
Maximum score	23
AIMS65 score	
Albumin <3.0 g/dL	1
INR >1.5	1
Altered mental status	1
SBP ≤90 mm Hg	1
Age >65 y	1
Maximum score	5
Rockall score	
Age, y[a]	
<60	0
60–79	1
>80	2
Shock[a]	
No shock	0
Pulse >100 bpm, SBP >100 mm Hg	1
SBP <100 mm Hg	2
Comorbidity[a]	
No major	0

(continued on next page)

Table 1 (continued)	
Risk Factor	Points
CHF, IHD, or major comorbidity	2
Renal failure, liver failure, or metastatic cancer	3
Diagnosis	
Mallory-Weiss tear or no lesion and no stigmata	0
All other diagnoses	1
GI malignancy	2
Evidence of bleeding	
No stigmata or dark spot on ulcer	0
Blood in upper GI tract, adherent clot, visible or spurting vessel	2
Maximum score	11

Abbreviations: bpm, beats per minute; BUN, blood urea nitrogen; CHF, congestive heart failure; GI, gastrointestinal; IHD, ischemic heart disease; INR, international normalized ratio; SBP, systolic blood pressure.

[a] Components of clinical or preendoscopic Rockall score.

superior to both the GBS and the preendoscopy Rockall score in predicting inhospital mortality, need for ICU admission, and LOS.[35] Notably, the GBS was superior to all other scores (including the full Rockall score) for predicting blood transfusion. Tang and colleagues[36] compared the performance of multiple risk assessment scores in an emergency department setting. Among 395 subjects, the AIMS65 score and GBS were superior to the preendoscopic Rockall score in predicting 30-day mortality. In a recent large, international, multicenter prospective study of 3012 subjects, comparing both preendoscopic (AIMS65, GBS, preendoscopic Rockall) and postendoscopic (full Rockall, Progetto Nazionale Emorragia Digestiva [PNED][37]) scoring systems, the GBS was superior to all other scores at predicting intervention (a composite endpoint of blood transfusion, endoscopy, interventional radiology, or surgery) or inpatient death, and superior to the preendoscopic Rockall and AIMS65 scores at predicting the need for endoscopic treatment.[38] The AIMS65 and PNED scores were superior compared with the GBS and preendoscopic Rockall scores in predicting 30-day mortality. Similar to earlier findings, a GBS score of 0 or 1 predicted survival without intervention (sensitivity 98.6% and specificity 34.6%), whereas a GBS greater than or equal to 7 predicted the need for endoscopic treatment (sensitivity 80%, specificity 57%). Thresholds of greater than or equal to 2 for AIMS65, greater than or equal to 4 for preendoscopic Rockall, and greater than or equal to 5 for full Rockall scores were optimal in predicting inhospital death.[38,39]

Although the use of these risk stratification systems are strongly encouraged in current guidelines, a 2014 nationwide study in the United States of 1402 emergency physicians, internists, and gastroenterologists revealed that only 53% had ever heard of and 30% had ever used a UGIB risk score.[40] Possible barriers to adherence include lack of knowledge because the literature on risk assessment in UGIB is primarily published in gastroenterology and endoscopy journals, as well as difficulty in recalling risk parameters and their corresponding scores.

Kumar and colleagues[41] postulated that the use of only 1 predictor, an increase in blood urea nitrogen (BUN) at 24 hours, may correlate with worse outcomes in nonvariceal UGIB similar to the way BUN does in acute pancreatitis because both clinical scenarios require aggressive volume resuscitation in their initial management. In a retrospective study of 357 subjects with UGIB, those with an increased BUN level at 24 hours compared with the BUN value at presentation were significantly more likely to experience a composite outcome (including inpatient death, rebleeding, need for surgery or radiologic intervention, or endoscopic reintervention), as well as inpatient mortality, compared with patients with a decreased or unchanged BUN. These data suggest that, in addition to prognostic information provided by other risk stratification scores, the use of a solitary clinical parameter, an increase in BUN at 24 hours, predicts worse outcomes in acute nonvariceal UGIB, likely as an indicator of inadequate fluid resuscitation.

NASOGASTRIC LAVAGE

NG intubation in patients with nonvariceal UGIB has been traditionally thought to provide diagnostic and prognostic information regarding the source and severity of gastrointestinal bleeding. However, its placement is not without risk, including severe patient discomfort. Singer and colleagues[42] evaluated 15 of the most common procedures performed in the emergency department and found that NG intubation was the most painful according to patients, even more so than abscess drainage, fracture reduction, or urethral catheterization. Although NG lavage has been associated with an earlier time to endoscopy, this does not affect clinical outcomes such as mortality, LOS, or need for surgery or transfusion.[43] Furthermore, a recent single-blind, prospective, randomized, noninferiority study of 280 subjects confirmed that routine NG tube placement and lavage did not improve the probability of finding a high-risk lesion on endoscopy, did not affect rebleeding or mortality rates, and was complicated by pain and bleeding nares in a quarter of subjects.[44] Due to its lack of patient benefits and its adverse events, including pain, current guidelines do not recommend routine NG tube placement or lavage in the early management of patients with suspected nonvariceal UGIB.

VIDEO CAPSULE ENDOSCOPY

VCE can be a useful noninvasive tool to identify which patients presenting with symptoms suggestive of UGIB may require hospitalization for high-risk lesions. Gralnek and colleagues[45] conducted a prospective study of 49 subjects in which VCE performed in the emergency department detected blood in the stomach at a significantly higher rate than NG tube aspiration (83.3% vs 33.3%, $P = .035$) and had a similar rate of identification of peptic or inflammatory lesions compared with upper endoscopy. VCE has also been shown to be more accurate than clinical scoring tools in predicting high-risk endoscopic stigmata and more cost-effective than GBS, NG lavage, or admit-all strategies in subjects with low-risk and moderate-risk UGIB.[46,47] In a prospective randomized controlled trial of 71 subjects, Sung and colleagues[48] found that use of VCE in the emergency department reduced hospital admission by nearly 80%, with no rebleeding or 30-day mortality in subjects who had a negative VCE study and were subsequently discharged. Although VCE is not currently included in guidelines for the initial management of UGIB, these studies suggest a possible future role in triage and risk stratification. However, further developments are needed, including the availability of a VCE designed specifically for evaluation of UGIB and decreases in costs.

TIMING OF ENDOSCOPY

Upper endoscopy is a critical aspect in the management of nonvariceal UGIB for both diagnosis and therapeutic intervention. Current guidelines recommend that endoscopy be performed within 24 hours of presentation[6,9,28]; however, the role of more urgent endoscopy remains controversial. In general, endoscopy performed within 12 hours of presentation identified more high-risk lesions but with no associated improvement in clinical outcomes, whereas endoscopy performed within 24 hours decreased the length of hospital stay and possibly the need for surgery without major complications (**Table 2**).

Immediate Endoscopy (<3 Hours)

In a randomized clinical trial, 110 subjects were assigned to receive immediate endoscopy (within 1–2 hours of presentation) versus elective endoscopy (within 48 hours).[49] Subjects who underwent immediate endoscopy were found to have a significantly shorter LOS (1 vs 2 days, $P = .001$) and lower hospitalization costs ($2068 vs $3662, $P<.001$). However, there were no significant differences in clinical outcomes, including mortality; recurrent bleeding; and the need for transfusion, surgery, or repeat endoscopy between the 2 groups. Similar results were found in a retrospective study of 81 subjects with peptic ulcer bleeding who underwent endoscopy within 3 hours versus 48 hours.[50] There was no benefit to immediate endoscopy with regard to mortality, rebleeding, surgery, or LOS compared with later endoscopy, despite a higher rate of detection of actively spurting peptic ulcers (19% vs 3%, $P = .022$) and need for endoscopic therapy (77% vs 47%, $P = .006$) in the early group.

Emergent Endoscopy (<12 Hours)

Eight studies have examined outcomes of endoscopy performed within 6 to 12 hours of presentation. In a prospective randomized controlled trial of UGIB from peptic ulcers, 325 subjects were assigned to endoscopy within 12 hours or endoscopy after 12 hours.[51] All subjects also underwent NG lavage and the aspirate was categorized as clear, coffee-ground, or bloody. In subjects with clear or coffee-ground aspirates, there were no significant differences in clinical outcomes, including mortality, between early and delayed endoscopy groups. However, in subjects with bloody NG aspirate, those who underwent emergent endoscopy had a decreased volume of blood transfused (450 mL vs 666 mL, $P<.001$) and shorter LOS (4 vs 14.5 days, $P<.001$).

In another randomized controlled trial of 93 subjects with hemodynamically stable UGIB, individuals were assigned to undergo either emergent endoscopy (within 6 hours) or elective endoscopy (within 48 hours).[52] No differences were found in clinical outcomes despite the emergent group having more high-risk endoscopic lesions (32% vs 20%, $P = .017$).

A retrospective study of 169 hemodynamically unstable subjects with nonvariceal UGIB evaluated the role of endoscopy within 6 hours versus 24 hours of admission.[53] Again, emergent endoscopy detected an increased rate of high-risk lesions (57% vs 37%, $P = .01$) and endoscopic treatment (53% vs 37%, $P = .04$); however, there were no differences between the groups in terms of mortality, rebleeding, or surgery. Importantly, although all subjects had abnormal vital signs at presentation, neither emergent nor standard groups had preendoscopic Rockall scores (3.2 and 3.3, respectively) that would suggest a high-risk outcome.

In another retrospective study, 189 subjects underwent endoscopy either within 8 hours or between 8 and 24 hours from time of admission.[54] As with previous studies, no significant differences were found between the 2 groups with regard to mortality, rebleeding, blood transfusion, or LOS. However, high-risk lesions, such as actively bleeding ulcers (19% vs 8%, $P = .03$) or visible vessels (34% vs 12%, $P<.01$), were more likely to be identified and subsequently treated (40% vs 15%, $P<.001$) in the emergent endoscopy group.

Table 2
Summary of results of selected articles on timing of endoscopy for nonvariceal upper gastrointestinal bleeding

Authors	Study Size	Upper Endoscopy Timing for Treatment Group	Upper Endoscopy Timing for Control Group	Treatment vs Control Group Outcomes			
				Death (%)	Rebleeding (%)	Surgery (%)	LOS (median, d)
Immediate endoscopy (<3 h)							
Lee et al,[49] 1999	110	≤2 h	≤48 h	0 vs 3.7	3.6 vs 5.6	3.6 vs 1.9	1 vs 2[a]
Schacher et al,[50] 2005	81	≤3 h	≤48 h	0 vs 0	14.0 vs 15.8	9.3 vs 7.9	5.1 vs 5.9
Emergent endoscopy (<12 h)							
Lin et al,[51] 1996[b]	107	≤12 h	>12 h	1.9 vs 1.9	5.7 vs 9.3	5.7 vs 7.4	—
Bjorkman et al,[52] 2004	93	≤6 h	≤48 h	0 vs 0	—	2.1 vs 2.2	3 vs 3
Targownik et al,[53] 2007	169	≤6 h	≤24 h	8 vs 6	9 vs 8	8 vs 2	4 vs 4
Tai et al,[54] 2007	189	≤8 h	≤24 h	1.1 vs 5.9	—	0 vs 0	5.1 vs 6.0
Ahn et al,[55] 2016	158	≤8 h	≤24 h	1.7 vs 2	6.7 vs 5.1	—	7.3 vs 9.1
Cho et al,[56] 2017[c]	961	≤6 h	≤24 h	1.6 vs 3.8[a]	11.4 vs 9.0	1.1 vs 0	6.7 vs 6.4
Kumar et al,[57] 2017[c]	361	≤12 h	>12 h	4 vs 1	11 vs 4[a]	4 vs 0[a]	4.3 vs 4
Early endoscopy (within 24 h)							
Cooper et al,[59] 1999	909	≤24 h	>24 h	3.8 vs 3.4	—	—	5.0 vs 6.4[a]
Cooper et al,[60] 2009	2592	≤1 d	>1 d	6.2 vs 7.3	—	1.2 vs 3.4[a]	4 vs 6[a]
Garg et al,[61] 2017	2066707	≤24 h	>24 h	3 vs 4.2[a]	—	—	4.6 vs 0.02[a]
Lim et al,[62] 2011[c]	97	≤13 h	>13 h	0 vs 44[a]	12.0 vs 14.9	0 vs 2.1	5.6 vs 19.5[a]

[a] Statistically significant.
[b] Subgroup analysis of patients with coffee-grounds or bloody aspirate on nasogastric lavage.
[c] Subgroup analysis of high-risk patients.

A retrospective study from Korea evaluated 158 subjects who presented with UGIB to the emergency department after hours (6 PM to 8 PM on weekdays and 1 PM Saturdays to 8 AM Mondays).[55] Among them, 50 subjects underwent endoscopy within 8 hours, whereas 98 received endoscopy within 24 hours. Again, there were no significant differences in primary hemostasis, rebleeding, and 30-day mortality between the 2 groups, though emergent endoscopy predicted a shorter LOS compared with later endoscopy (7.8 days vs 10.6 days, $P = .04$).

More recently, a retrospective evaluation of 961 subjects with higher risk UGIB (GBS >7) found that emergent endoscopy (within 6 hours) was associated with a lower 28-day mortality, the number of transfused packed red blood cells, and the need for intervention and embolization compared with later endoscopy (within 48 hours).[56] There were no differences between the groups in terms of rebleeding, ICU admission, vasopressor use, or LOS.

To investigate whether patients admitted with lower risk (GBS <12) versus higher risk (GBS ≥12) nonvariceal UGIB have different outcomes depending on urgency of endoscopy, a retrospective study was performed with 361 subjects.[57] Overall, subjects who underwent urgent endoscopy had a greater than 5-fold increased risk of reaching a composite outcome of death, rebleeding, or need for surgery. Radiologic or repeat endoscopic intervention (unadjusted odds ratio [OR] 5.6, $P<.001$) was primarily driven by lower risk subjects. A large Danish cohort study of 12,601 subjects with peptic ulcer bleeding also evaluated the relationship between timing of endoscopy and mortality stratified by preendoscopic risk as defined hemodynamic stability and an American Society of Anesthesiologists (ASA) score.[58] In subjects who were hemodynamically stable with an ASA score of 1 to 2, there was no association between timing of endoscopy and mortality; however, a subgroup analysis of subjects presenting with peptic ulcer bleeding outside the hospital showed that endoscopy within 24 hours was associated with reduced inhospital mortality. In subjects who were hemodynamically stable with an ASA score of 3 to 5, there was a U-shaped association between timing of endoscopy and mortality in which the nadir of inhospital mortality occurred when endoscopy was performed between 12 and 36 hours from the time of admission or from the time of development of symptoms. Endoscopy during this time interval was associated with a significant reduction in inhospital mortality (OR 0.48, $P<.001$) compared with endoscopy performed outside this time interval. In subjects with hemodynamic instability, the association between timing of endoscopy and mortality was less clear, regardless of ASA score. The investigators hypothesized that performing endoscopy between 6 and 24 hours could be associated with optimal outcome and found that subjects who underwent endoscopy during this interval experienced a lower inhospital mortality (OR 0.73, $P = .035$), as well as 30-day mortality (OR 0.66, $P = .025$), compared with subjects who underwent endoscopy outside this time period. These studies are the first to suggest that earlier endoscopy may in fact pose potential harm, including in subjects who have a low preendoscopic risk assessment.

Early Endoscopy (Within 24 Hours)

In a retrospective study of 909 subjects across 13 different hospitals, clinical outcomes were compared between those who received endoscopy within 24 hours and those who received endoscopy after 24 hours.[59] There was no significant difference in mortality, rebleeding, or need for surgery; however, early endoscopy was associated with a decrease in LOS (5 vs 6.4 days, $P<.001$). In subgroup analysis, subjects with high-risk lesions who underwent endoscopic treatment had a decreased rate of recurrent bleeding and surgery.

A large nationwide retrospective study evaluated 2592 subjects who underwent endoscopy within 1 day of presentation versus elective endoscopy after 1 day.[60] Again, there was no mortality benefit from endoscopy within 24 hours; however, early endoscopy did confer a similar decrease in LOS and need for surgery compared with the elective group.

A population-based study using the National Inpatient Sample database evaluated 2,066,707 patients with UGIB (based on discharge diagnostic codes).[61] Among these patients, 84% underwent upper endoscopy during their admission. Patients who had early endoscopy within 24 hours had a significantly lower mortality rate compared with patients who had delayed endoscopy after 24 hours or patients who had no endoscopy at all (3% vs 4.2% vs 8.5%, $P<.001$). On multivariate analysis, patients with delayed endoscopy were 1.4 times more likely to die ($P<.001$), hospitalized 3.7 days longer ($P<.001$), and incurred $28,024.62 more in hospital costs ($P<.001$) compared with subjects who underwent early endoscopy.

Endoscopy Timing Using Risk Stratification

Lim and colleagues[62] prospectively enrolled 934 subjects with nonvariceal UGIB and retrospectively calculated their GBS at presentation to stratify subjects into low-risk (GBS <12) and high-risk (GBS ≥12) groups. In lower risk subjects, the timing of endoscopy was not associated with inpatient mortality; however, in high-risk subjects, the timing of endoscopy was the only significant predictor of mortality after adjusting for multiple confounders (adjusted OR 1.09, 95% CI 1.02–1.17), whereas all deaths occurred in subjects who had endoscopy after 13 hours. This study was the first to identify a potential mortality benefit for urgent endoscopy in high-risk subjects. It is possible; however, that high-risk subjects who had delayed endoscopy required longer initial resuscitation and were therefore more likely to die.

In a prospective, multicenter study (published as an abstract), 3207 subjects with nonvariceal UGIB were stratified as low-risk, medium-rick, or high-risk of death based on 10 clinical parameters identified through logistic regression, including age older than 80 years, inhospital bleeding, hematemesis, hypotension (systolic blood pressure <100 mm Hg, diastolic blood pressure <60 mm Hg), heart rate greater than 100 beats per minute, and hemoglobin less than 7 g/dL, as well as the presence of renal failure, cirrhosis or neoplasia.[63] Timing of endoscopy was categorized into 3 intervals: within 6 hours, between 7 and 12 hours, and between 13 and 24 hours. In low-risk and medium-risk subjects, mortality was not significantly different across the 3 time intervals ($P = .192$ and .678, respectively). In subjects at high risk, mortality was lowest in those who underwent endoscopy between 13 and 24 hours (3.93%) compared with those who underwent endoscopy between 7 and 12 hours (6%) and those who received endoscopy within 6 hours (5.74%, $P = .001$). These conflicting results suggest that additional evidence is needed to evaluate the use of risk stratification in determining the most appropriate time for endoscopy.

SUMMARY

The inhospital mortality from nonvariceal UGIB has improved with recent advances in medical and endoscopic therapies. Initial management includes placement of 2 large-bore IV catheters, adequate fluid resuscitation, hemodynamic monitoring, PPI therapy, and a restrictive blood transfusion strategy. Risk stratification scores can help triage the severity of bleeding and provide prognostic information. Upper endoscopy is recommended within 24 hours of patient presentation. However, patients with very low risk, based on several risk stratification scores, may be effectively treated as outpatients. Emergent endoscopy within 12 hours has generally not been shown to significantly improve clinical outcomes, including mortality, rebleeding, or need for surgery, despite an increased use of endoscopic treatment, although there may be a benefit to emergent endoscopy in patients with evidence of ongoing active bleeding.

REFERENCES

1. Tielleman T, Bujanda D, Cryer B. Epidemiology and risk factors for upper gastrointestinal bleeding. Gastrointest Endosc Clin N Am 2015;25(3):415–28.
2. Abougergi MS, Travis AC, Saltzman JR. The in-hospital mortality rate for upper GI hemorrhage has decreased over 2 decades in the United States: a nationwide analysis. Gastrointest Endosc 2015;81(4):882–8.e1.
3. Rotondano G. Epidemiology and diagnosis of acute nonvariceal upper gastrointestinal bleeding. Gastroenterol Clin North Am 2014;43(4):643–63.
4. Tsoi KK, Ma TK, Sung JJ. Endoscopy for upper gastrointestinal bleeding: how urgent is it? Nat Rev Gastroenterol Hepatol 2009;6(8):463–9.
5. Hwang JH, Fisher DA, Ben-Menachem T, et al. The role of endoscopy in the management of acute non-variceal upper GI bleeding. Gastrointest Endosc 2012; 75(6):1132–8.
6. Laine L, Jensen DM. Management of patients with ulcer bleeding. Am J Gastroenterol 2012;107(3):345–60 [quiz: 361].
7. Sung JJ, Chan FK, Chen M, et al. Asia-Pacific Working Group consensus on nonvariceal upper gastrointestinal bleeding. Gut 2011;60(9):1170–7.
8. Dworzynski K, Pollit V, Kelsey A, et al. Management of acute upper gastrointestinal bleeding: summary of NICE guidance. BMJ 2012;344:e3412.
9. Gralnek IM, Dumonceau JM, Kuipers EJ, et al. Diagnosis and management of nonvariceal upper gastrointestinal hemorrhage: European Society of Gastrointestinal Endoscopy (ESGE) Guideline. Endoscopy 2015;47(10):a1–46.
10. Kumar NL, Travis AC, Saltzman JR. Initial management and timing of endoscopy in nonvariceal upper GI bleeding. Gastrointest Endosc 2016;84(1):10–7.
11. Hayat U, Lee PJ, Ullah H, et al. Association of prophylactic endotracheal intubation in critically ill patients with upper GI bleeding and cardiopulmonary unplanned events. Gastrointest Endosc 2017;86(3):500–9.e1.
12. Worden JC, Hanna KS. Optimizing proton pump inhibitor therapy for treatment of nonvariceal upper gastrointestinal bleeding. Am J Health Syst Pharm 2017;74(3): 109–16.
13. Leontiadis GI, Sharma VK, Howden CW. Systematic review and meta-analysis of proton pump inhibitor therapy in peptic ulcer bleeding. BMJ 2005;330(7491):568.
14. Lin HJ, Lo WC, Lee FY, et al. A prospective randomized comparative trial showing that omeprazole prevents rebleeding in patients with bleeding peptic ulcer after successful endoscopic therapy. Arch Intern Med 1998;158(1):54–8.
15. Khuroo MS, Yattoo GN, Javid G, et al. A comparison of omeprazole and placebo for bleeding peptic ulcer. N Engl J Med 1997;336(15):1054–8.
16. Lau JY, Sung JJ, Lee KK, et al. Effect of intravenous omeprazole on recurrent bleeding after endoscopic treatment of bleeding peptic ulcers. N Engl J Med 2000;343(5):310–6.
17. Schaffalitzky de Muckadell OB, Havelund T, Harling H, et al. Effect of omeprazole on the outcome of endoscopically treated bleeding peptic ulcers. Randomized double-blind placebo-controlled multicentre study. Scand J Gastroenterol 1997; 32(4):320–7.

18. Sung JJ, Chan FK, Lau JY, et al. The effect of endoscopic therapy in patients receiving omeprazole for bleeding ulcers with nonbleeding visible vessels or adherent clots: a randomized comparison. Ann Intern Med 2003;139(4):237–43.

19. Lau JY, Leung WK, Wu JC, et al. Omeprazole before endoscopy in patients with gastrointestinal bleeding. N Engl J Med 2007;356(16):1631–40.

20. Laine L, McQuaid KR. Endoscopic therapy for bleeding ulcers: an evidence-based approach based on meta-analyses of randomized controlled trials. Clin Gastroenterol Hepatol 2009;7(1):33–47 [quiz: 31–2].

21. Sachar H, Vaidya K, Laine L. Intermittent vs continuous proton pump inhibitor therapy for high-risk bleeding ulcers: a systematic review and meta-analysis. JAMA Intern Med 2014;174(11):1755–62.

22. Lu Y, Adam V, Teich V, et al. Timing or dosing of intravenous proton pump inhibitors in acute upper gastrointestinal bleeding has low impact on costs. Am J Gastroenterol 2016;111(10):1389–98.

23. Hebert PC, Wells G, Blajchman MA, et al. A multicenter, randomized, controlled clinical trial of transfusion requirements in critical care. Transfusion Requirements in Critical Care Investigators, Canadian Critical Care Trials Group. N Engl J Med 1999;340(6):409–17.

24. Hearnshaw SA, Logan RF, Palmer KR, et al. Outcomes following early red blood cell transfusion in acute upper gastrointestinal bleeding. Aliment Pharmacol Ther 2010;32(2):215–24.

25. Halland M, Young M, Fitzgerald MN, et al. Characteristics and outcomes of upper gastrointestinal hemorrhage in a tertiary referral hospital. Dig Dis Sci 2010;55(12):3430–5.

26. Villanueva C, Colomo A, Bosch A, et al. Transfusion strategies for acute upper gastrointestinal bleeding. N Engl J Med 2013;368(1):11–21.

27. Odutayo A, Desborough MJ, Trivella M, et al. Restrictive versus liberal blood transfusion for gastrointestinal bleeding: a systematic review and meta-analysis of randomised controlled trials. Lancet Gastroenterol Hepatol 2017;2(5):354–60.

28. Barkun AN, Bardou M, Kuipers EJ, et al. International consensus recommendations on the management of patients with nonvariceal upper gastrointestinal bleeding. Ann Intern Med 2010;152(2):101–13.

29. Blatchford O, Murray WR, Blatchford M. A risk score to predict need for treatment for upper-gastrointestinal haemorrhage. Lancet 2000;356(9238):1318–21.

30. Stanley AJ, Ashley D, Dalton HR, et al. Outpatient management of patients with low-risk upper-gastrointestinal haemorrhage: multicentre validation and prospective evaluation. Lancet 2009;373(9657):42–7.

31. Srygley FD, Gerardo CJ, Tran T, et al. Does this patient have a severe upper gastrointestinal bleed? JAMA 2012;307(10):1072–9.

32. Saltzman JR, Tabak YP, Hyett BH, et al. A simple risk score accurately predicts in-hospital mortality, length of stay, and cost in acute upper GI bleeding. Gastrointest Endosc 2011;74(6):1215–24.

33. Abougergi MS, Charpentier JP, Bethea E, et al. A prospective, multicenter study of the AIMS65 score compared with the glasgow-blatchford score in predicting upper gastrointestinal hemorrhage outcomes. J Clin Gastroenterol 2016;50(6):464–9.

34. Rockall TA, Logan RF, Devlin HB, et al. Risk assessment after acute upper gastrointestinal haemorrhage. Gut 1996;38(3):316–21.

35. Robertson M, Majumdar A, Boyapati R, et al. Risk stratification in acute upper GI bleeding: comparison of the AIMS65 score with the Glasgow-Blatchford and Rockall scoring systems. Gastrointest Endosc 2016;83(6):1151–60.

36. Tang Y, Shen J, Zhang F, et al. Comparison of four scoring systems used to predict mortality in patients with acute upper gastrointestinal bleeding in the emergency room. Am J Emerg Med 2018;36(1):27–32.

37. Contreras-Omana R, Alfaro-Reynoso JA, Cruz-Chavez CE, et al. The Progetto Nazionale Emorragia Digestiva (PNED) system vs. the Rockall score as mortality predictors in patients with nonvariceal upper gastrointestinal bleeding: a multicenter prospective study. Rev Gastroenterol Mex 2017;82(2):123–8.

38. Stanley AJ, Laine L, Dalton HR, et al. Comparison of risk scoring systems for patients presenting with upper gastrointestinal bleeding: international multicentre prospective study. BMJ 2017;356:i6432.

39. Hyett BH, Abougergi MS, Charpentier JP, et al. The AIMS65 score compared with the Glasgow-Blatchford score in predicting outcomes in upper GI bleeding. Gastrointest Endosc 2013;77(4):551–7.

40. Liang PS, Saltzman JR. A national survey on the initial management of upper gastrointestinal bleeding. J Clin Gastroenterol 2014;48(10):e93–8.

41. Kumar NL, Claggett BL, Cohen AJ, et al. Association between an increase in blood urea nitrogen at 24 hours and worse outcomes in acute nonvariceal upper GI bleeding. Gastrointest Endosc 2017;86(6):1022–7.e1.

42. Singer AJ, Richman PB, Kowalska A, et al. Comparison of patient and practitioner assessments of pain from commonly performed emergency department procedures. Ann Emerg Med 1999;33(6):652–8.

43. Huang ES, Karsan S, Kanwal F, et al. Impact of nasogastric lavage on outcomes in acute GI bleeding. Gastrointest Endosc 2011;74(5):971–80.

44. Rockey DC, Ahn C, de Melo SW Jr. Randomized pragmatic trial of nasogastric tube placement in patients with upper gastrointestinal tract bleeding. J Investig Med 2017;65(4):759–64.

45. Gralnek IM, Ching JY, Maza I, et al. Capsule endoscopy in acute upper gastrointestinal hemorrhage: a prospective cohort study. Endoscopy 2013;45(1):12–9.

46. Gutkin E, Shalomov A, Hussain SA, et al. Pillcam ESO (®) is more accurate than clinical scoring systems in risk stratifying emergency room patients with acute upper gastrointestinal bleeding. Therap Adv Gastroenterol 2013;6(3):193–8.

47. Meltzer AC, Ward MJ, Gralnek IM, et al. The cost-effectiveness analysis of video capsule endoscopy compared to other strategies to manage acute upper gastrointestinal hemorrhage in the ED. Am J Emerg Med 2014;32(8):823–32.

48. Sung JJ, Tang RS, Ching JY, et al. Use of capsule endoscopy in the emergency department as a triage of patients with GI bleeding. Gastrointest Endosc 2016; 84(6):907–13.

49. Lee JG, Turnipseed S, Romano PS, et al. Endoscopy-based triage significantly reduces hospitalization rates and costs of treating upper GI bleeding: a randomized controlled trial. Gastrointest Endosc 1999;50(6):755–61.

50. Schacher GM, Lesbros-Pantoflickova D, Ortner MA, et al. Is early endoscopy in the emergency room beneficial in patients with bleeding peptic ulcer? A "fortuitously controlled" study. Endoscopy 2005;37(4):324–8.

51. Lin HJ, Wang K, Perng CL, et al. Early or delayed endoscopy for patients with peptic ulcer bleeding. A prospective randomized study. J Clin Gastroenterol 1996;22(4):267–71.

52. Bjorkman DJ, Zaman A, Fennerty MB, et al. Urgent vs. elective endoscopy for acute non-variceal upper-GI bleeding: an effectiveness study. Gastrointest Endosc 2004;60(1):1–8.

53. Targownik LE, Murthy S, Keyvani L, et al. The role of rapid endoscopy for high-risk patients with acute nonvariceal upper gastrointestinal bleeding. Can J Gastroenterol 2007;21(7):425–9.

54. Tai CM, Huang SP, Wang HP, et al. High-risk ED patients with nonvariceal upper gastrointestinal hemorrhage undergoing emergency or urgent endoscopy: a retrospective analysis. Am J Emerg Med 2007;25(3):273–8.

55. Ahn DW, Park YS, Lee SH, et al. Clinical outcome of acute nonvariceal upper gastrointestinal bleeding after hours: the role of urgent endoscopy. Korean J Intern Med 2016;31(3):470–8.

56. Cho SH, Lee YS, Kim YJ, et al. Outcomes and role of urgent endoscopy in high-risk patients with acute nonvariceal gastrointestinal bleeding. Clin Gastroenterol Hepatol 2018;16(3):370–7.

57. Kumar NL, Cohen AJ, Nayor J, et al. Timing of upper endoscopy influences outcomes in patients with acute nonvariceal upper GI bleeding. Gastrointest Endosc 2017;85(5):945–52.e1.

58. Laursen SB, Leontiadis GI, Stanley AJ, et al. Relationship between timing of endoscopy and mortality in patients with peptic ulcer bleeding: a nationwide cohort study. Gastrointest Endosc 2017;85(5):936–44.e3.

59. Cooper GS, Chak A, Way LE, et al. Early endoscopy in upper gastrointestinal hemorrhage: associations with recurrent bleeding, surgery, and length of hospital stay. Gastrointest Endosc 1999;49(2):145–52.

60. Cooper GS, Kou TD, Wong RC. Use and impact of early endoscopy in elderly patients with peptic ulcer hemorrhage: a population-based analysis. Gastrointest Endosc 2009;70(2):229–35.

61. Garg SK, Anugwom C, Campbell J, et al. Early esophagogastroduodenoscopy is associated with better Outcomes in upper gastrointestinal bleeding: a nationwide study. Endosc Int open 2017;5(5):E376–e386.

62. Lim LG, Ho KY, Chan YH, et al. Urgent endoscopy is associated with lower mortality in high-risk but not low-risk nonvariceal upper gastrointestinal bleeding. Endoscopy 2011;43(4):300–6.

63. Marmo R, Del Piano M, Rotondano G, et al. Mortality from nonvariceal upper gastrointestinal bleeding: is it time to differentiate the timing of endoscopy? Gastrointest Endosc 2011;73(4S):AB224.

Endotherapy of Peptic Ulcer Bleeding

Debbie Troland, MB ChB, MRCP, Adrian Stanley, MD, FRCP*

KEYWORDS

- Nonvariceal upper GI hemorrhage • Peptic ulcer • Duodenal ulcer • Gastric ulcer
- Endoscopic therapy • Peptic ulcer bleeding

KEY POINTS

- Ulcers should be assessed and managed according to the Forrest classification. Forrest Ia, Ib, and IIa should receive endoscopic therapy.
- Ulcers with adherent clot should have attempted clot removal, then be considered for endoscopic therapy depending on findings.
- Epinephrine injection should not be used as monotherapy. Thermal therapy (or sclerosant or adhesive injection) together with epinephrine can be used.
- Mechanical therapy with clips can be used alone or together with epinephrine injection.
- Routine second look endoscopy after endoscopic therapy for bleeding ulcers is not recommended, but has a role in selected higher risk patients.

INTRODUCTION

Peptic ulcers account for 28% to 59% of nonvariceal upper gastrointestinal (GI) hemorrhage with duodenal ulcers responsible for 17% to 37% and gastric ulcers 11% to 24%.[1] Peptic ulcer disease has reduced in prevalence, probably owing to improved nonsteroidal antiinflammatory drug prescribing practice, increased testing, and treatment of *Helicobacter pylori* infection in addition to more widespread use of proton pump inhibitors. However bleeding from peptic ulcers continues to result in significant morbidity and mortality, with the latter reported at 2% to 11%.[2] Mortality for inpatients with upper GI bleeding is higher, owing to the increased comorbidities and older age of these patients.[3]

Over the years, endoscopic techniques and therapies have improved the management of peptic ulcer bleeding, with endotherapy becoming more accessible and technologically advanced. A 2007audit of upper GI bleeding in the UK reported data on 6750 patients, 36% of whom had peptic ulcer bleeding.[3] Outcomes were compared

Disclosure Statement: The authors have no competing interests to declare.
Gastrointestinal Unit, Glasgow Royal Infirmary, Walton Building, Castle Street, Glasgow G4 0SF, UK
* Corresponding author.
E-mail address: adrian.stanley@ggc.scot.nhs.uk

Gastrointest Endoscopy Clin N Am 28 (2018) 277–289
https://doi.org/10.1016/j.giec.2018.02.002 **giendo.theclinics.com**
1052-5157/18/Crown Copyright © 2018 Published by Elsevier Inc. All rights reserved.

with an earlier UK audit in 1993 and found improvements in rebleeding rates, need for surgical intervention, and mortality. The reduction in surgery rates from greater than 20% in the 1970s to less than 2% in the 2007 audit suggests that the development and widespread use of therapeutic endoscopy over this period has been a major factor in the reduced need for surgery.[3]

The increased availability of trained GI endoscopists and related staff allows earlier diagnosis, endoscopic therapy and decisions on management. During the initial years of endotherapy, patients were treated with injection of epinephrine into and around the bleeding point as monotherapy. As technology advanced, the injection of sclerosants and adhesives and the use of thermal and mechanical techniques were introduced, followed by the more recent use of new hemostatic techniques.

Many larger hospitals now offer a 24-hour upper GI bleeding service whereby patients presenting with an acute upper GI bleed can undergo endoscopy within 24 hours, with urgent endoscopy undertaken if patients present with major bleeding resulting in hemodynamic instability. Units often have access to multiple modalities for endotherapy and ideally will also have access to interventional radiology techniques and surgery for the small proportion of patients in whom endoscopic techniques fail to control bleeding. In this article, we discuss the modalities currently available for endoscopic therapy in peptic ulcer bleeding and review the evidence and current guidelines for their use.

ENDOSCOPIC ASSESSMENT

When endoscopy is carried out in patients with acute upper GI bleeding it is important to have a standardized strategy for classifying bleeding lesions.[4] The Forrest classification of stigmata of recent hemorrhage was developed around 40 years ago as a method to classify lesions and helps to stratify the risk of further bleeding and identify the treatment strategy[2,5] (**Table 1**). It has stood the test of time and is still widely used today, both in clinical practice and research studies. It aims to identify stigmata of recent hemorrhage and give prognostic information on the risk of rebleeding and mortality, as well as the need for endoscopic intervention versus medical therapy. It can guide decisions on whether the patient can be discharged from hospital and can help with decisions regarding the level of in-patient care when this is required.[2]

Table 1
Forrest classification

Forrest Classification	Description	Prevalence (n = 2401)	Further Bleeding Rate (n = 2994), Mean Rate (Range)[a]	Mortality (n = 1387), Mean Rate (Range)[a]
Ia	Spurting hemorrhage	12%	55% (17%–100%)	11% (0%–23%)
Ib	Oozing hemorrhage			
IIa	Nonbleeding visible vessel	8%	43% (0%–81%)	11% (0%–21%)
IIb	Adherent clot	8%	22% (14%–36%)	7% (0%–10%)
IIc	Flat pigmented spot	16%	10% (0%–13%)	3% (0%–10%)
III	Clean ulcer	55%	5% (0%–10%)	2% (0%–3%)

[a] Figures in prospective trials without endoscopy therapy.

Adapted from Laine L, Jensen DM. Management of patients with ulcer bleeding. Am J Gastroenterol 2012;107:345–60.

The trials assessing rebleeding in patients with peptic ulcer disease have all consistently shown that Forrest Ia, Ib, and IIa lesions are an independent risk factor for persistent bleeding or rebleeding and should, therefore, receive endotherapy.[1,2,5–9] This practice is accepted and recommended by American, British, European, and international guidelines.[1,2,8,9] Forrest Ia and Ib lesions have rebleeding and mortality rates of 55% and 11%, with Forrest IIa lesions having rebleeding and mortality of 43% and 11%, respectively.[10]

A metaanalysis of patients with actively bleeding lesions when comparing endoscopic therapy versus no endoscopic therapy report a significant decrease in rebleeding when endoscopic therapy is applied, with a number needed to treat of only 2.[6] For nonbleeding visible vessels (Forrest IIa), the number needed to treat to prevent rebleeding was 5. The need for urgent intervention and surgery was also significantly decreased in these patients.

Forrest IIc and III lesions have been consistently found to be associated with a low risk of rebleeding, at 10% and 5%, respectively. Mortality for patients with these lesions is also low at 3% and 2%, respectively.[10] Therefore, current guidelines recommend medical therapy alone for these lesions, with endoscopic intervention not required. Patients with Forrest IIc and III lesions may also be considered for early discharge from hospital given their low risk of poor outcome.

There is some controversy surrounding the assessment and management of Forrest IIb lesions—ulcers with adherent clot. Studies have shown conflicting and varied outcomes. The reported risk of rebleeding in IIb lesions varies between 8% and 36%.[11] A metaanalysis of 6 trials assessing management of patients with adherent clots suggested there was a significant advantage of endotherapy plus medical therapy compared with medical therapy alone with regard to rebleeding and need for surgical intervention, although there was no difference in duration of hospital stay, transfusion requirement, or mortality.[11] Conversely, a separate metaanalysis of 75 studies showed no benefit from endoscopic therapy for adherent clots and commented on the markedly variable results among published trials.[6] The variability is probably explained by poor interobserver agreement on what constitutes an adherent clot, because this can be difficult to distinguish from a small visible vessel or flat pigmented spot. It could also be explained by variable attempts to dislodge the clot, which can range from gentle washing with syringe irrigation alone, to more vigorous irrigation with a water pump device, to mechanical clot removal using a forceps or a snare.

A commonly used strategy for dealing with an adherent clot is to vigorously wash the clot, aiming to remove the clot and more accurately assess the underlying ulcer base for stigmata of bleeding. Circumferential injection of dilute epinephrine (eg, 1:10,000) should be used before clot removal. This approach may upgrade or downgrade the classification of the lesion and allow appropriate therapy. Vigorous irrigation has been shown to successfully expose the underlying stigmata in 26% to 43% of cases and reveals high-risk stigmata in 10%.[9] For clots that remain adherent, rebleeding has been reported in 0% to 35% patients.[9] Given the lack of clear benefit and the potential risks of causing or aggravating bleeding, there may be subgroups in which aggressive clot removal is less appealing, such as lesions on the posterior wall of the duodenum and lesser curvature of the stomach. These areas are more technically challenging to view and apply endotherapy and often involve larger caliber vessels.

However, it is also important to consider that the benefits of endoscopic therapy may be greater in those at higher risk of poor outcomes, such as older patients, inpatients, and those with significant comorbidities. To conclude, a pragmatic strategy for adherent clots is to wash the clot away to further characterize the lesion and consider endoscopic therapy if there is underlying high-risk endoscopic stigmata of hemorrhage. It is also important to use clinical judgment with regard to the risks and benefits of aggressive clot removal on a case-by-case basis.

Endoscopic diagnosis of an ulcer is based on good visualization and interpretation of the image by the endoscopist. The main drawback of the Forrest classification is that studies have shown that there is significant interobserver variability with regard to the classification of lesions. One study asked a panel of 14 international experts to classify 100 ulcers using video-clips of endoscopy and reported disagreement in more than one-third of cases.[12] This finding implies that many patients may not be given endoscopic therapy when other experts would consider it appropriate.

Given that the Forrest classification is 40 years old, it is important to ensure that this tool remains valid for current practice. In 2014, de Groot and colleagues[7] performed a study that aimed to assess whether this classification remains useful for the prediction of rebleeding and mortality in peptic ulcer bleeding, and to assess whether it could be simplified. They evaluated the Forrest classification in 397 patients and reported outcomes. The authors found that it was still a useful classification for predicting recurrence of bleeding in peptic ulcers. Interestingly, the risk of rebleeding was similar to that in the 1970s despite the wide use of proton pump inhibitor therapy and advances in endoscopic therapy. The classification seemed to be more reliable for gastric than duodenal ulcers, which may be owing to the location of gastric ulcers being generally easier to visualize and to apply endoscopic therapy. However, they found that the Forrest classification did not predict mortality. They also noted the importance of differentiating between spurting and oozing hemorrhage and suggested the possibility of simplifying the classification into high risk (Forrest Ia), increased risk (Forrest Ib-IIc), and low risk (Forrest III). This may help to decrease interobserver variability in categorizing lesions, but more data are required to confirm the clinical usefulness of this approach.

Ulcer size is another endoscopic predictor of poor outcome.[1] Ulcers with a diameter of greater than 2 cm are more difficult to treat and less amenable to therapy with mechanical clips or other endoscopic therapies compared with smaller ulcers. Ulcers located on the posterior wall of the duodenum or lesser curve of the stomach are also difficult to view and technically difficult to treat endoscopically.

ENDOSCOPIC THERAPIES
Injection Therapy

Epinephrine is commonly used and is injected into the surrounding tissue of a high-risk lesion via a catheter fed through the working channel of the endoscope. When the catheter is in an appropriate position, the needle can be extended and epinephrine injected. Epinephrine should be diluted with normal saline to a dose of 1:10,000 or 1:20,000.[1] Generally, 0.5 to 2.0 mL of solution is be injected at a time, in quadrants around the ulcer base.[13] The aim is to produce a tamponade effect as well as local vasoconstriction to minimize local blood flow. A study assessing the association between total volume of epinephrine injection and outcome showed that injection of between 13 and 20 mL total volume significantly improved rebleeding rates when compared with smaller volumes.[14]

The injection of sclerosants has also been used to disrupt blood flow. These include ethanol, ethanolamine, and polidocanol. The aim is to cause direct injury to the tissue and thrombosis of the vessels to stop bleeding. Sclerosant therapy has been shown to be effective in reducing further bleeding, the need for surgery, and mortality.[6] However, their use is relatively limited owing to concerns about causing tissue necrosis, pancreatitis, and perforation, meaning that only small volumes of 0.1 to 0.2 mL aliquots with a maximum of 1.2 mL should be administered. The injection of sclerosant as monotherapy is not recommended.[1,2]

Tissue adhesives are another injectable modality. These include thrombin, fibrin, and cyanoacrylate glues. They are injected to create a primary seal at the bleeding site to stop active bleeding and prevent rebleeding. However, reported adverse events include perforation and damage to the endoscope.

Thermal

A heater probe is a contact thermal device that uses both the tamponade effect of direct pressure and heat to cause coagulation of blood vessels via the constriction of vessels, activation of the coagulation cascade, and tissue edema and coagulation. Heater probes are available in 7F and 10F sizes and have a Teflon-coated hollow aluminum cylinder with an inner heating coil and thermocoupling device at the tip of the probe, which is fed through the working channel of the endoscope. This maintains a constant energy output that is usually delivered at 15 to 30 J. The device is controlled by the endoscopist via a foot pedal that can be used for delivering energy as well as having the added benefit of a water jet device for irrigation. A heater probe is commonly used, because it is relatively inexpensive and portable, and has been shown to be efficacious and safe.[15]

Bipolar electrocautery is another contact thermal device. This device generates heat indirectly by the passage of an electrical current through the tissues. A local electrical circuit is completed between 2 electrodes on the tip of the device, with the current flowing through the tissue causing coagulation of vessels. When the tissue is desiccated, the electrical conductivity decreases, which limits the extent of tissue injury and depth and improves safety. Bipolar electrocautery devices are also activated via an endoscopist-controlled foot pedal. Settings of between 15 and 20 W are generally applied in approximately 8- to 10-second applications (tamponade station) to achieve hemostasis.[1,16] Bipolar eletrocoagulation has been shown to be more effective than no endoscopic therapy, with reduced rebleeding rates, need for surgery, and mortality.[2]

Argon plasma coagulation (APC) is a noncontact thermal modality that uses a high-frequency monopolar current conducted through a stream of ionized gas to coagulate superficial tissue. The coagulation depth depends on the power setting, gas flow rate, duration of application, and distance from the tissue. The tissue closest to the electrode is affected whether en face or tangential, which can be helpful in certain anatomic locations. The distance between the probe and tissue should be between 2 and 8 mm with power settings of 40 to 50 W, flow rate of 0.8 L/min, and applications between 0.5 and 2.0 seconds duration.[16,17] Despite the mechanisms to limit depth of coagulation, deep tissue injury can occur. A small randomized trial compared APC with heater probe for endoscopic hemostasis in bleeding ulcers and reported no difference in outcomes.[18] The APC delivery system is more complex and costly when compared with the standard heater probe and, therefore, is less widely used.

Endoscopic laser coagulation is another noncontact modality for management of bleeding peptic ulcer disease. An Nd:YAG laser is applied via the channel of an endoscope with the tip positioned 5 to 10 mm from the ulcer and the beam directed at the site of bleeding. There should be 75-W energy administered in 0.5-second pulses. In a trial assessing this modality for bleeding peptic ulcers, patients were treated with either standard medical treatment alone or standard medical treatment combined with laser photocoagulation.[19] Although laser therapy arrested active bleeding, there was no effect on transfusion requirement, surgical intervention, rebleeding, or mortality. Another trial assessing Nd:YAG laser showed benefit in rebleeding rates when compared with no endoscopic therapy.[20] However, the laser delivery unit is large and cumbersome, requires special electrical and water supplies, is costly compared with other methods of thermal coagulation, and is today an historical footnote in the treatment of peptic ulcer bleeding.

Mechanical

Mechanical hemostasis can be achieved by application of "through-the-scope" endoscopic clips. These are devices that are passed through the endoscope working channel, with the clip deployed directly onto and around the bleeding site to compress blood flow. There are several types of clips available that differ in opening width and jaw length, as well as their ability to rotate and to reopen after partial closure[21,22] (**Table 2**).

The clips are encased within a catheter that is passed through the endoscope. The clip is then unsheathed and positioned in the desirable area with a "plunger" handle used to open and close the clip. Rotation allows easier orientation of the clip to the optimal position for deployment. Newer clips have the option to be opened, partially closed and reopened if needed before final deployment, whereas others are permanently deployed upon initial clip closure. Once applied, the clips tend to slough off after several days. A clip is also now available that allows 3 clip applications without changing the applicator.[22] A clip with 3 branches (TriClip, Cook Medical, Bloomington, IN) was previously developed; however, evidence suggested inferior outcomes for primary hemostasis and rebleeding rates.[22]

Mechanical hemostasis aims to offer permanent closure of smaller vessels; however, blood vessels that are greater than 2 mm are more difficult to treat with conventional clips.[22] Technical factors can adversely affect clip placement, including access to lesions in challenging anatomic positions such as the posterior wall of the duodenum, proximal stomach, and lesser curve. Applying a clip to a very fibrotic ulcer base can also be difficult. However, clip application in peptic ulcer bleeding is generally safe and not associated with significant tissue injury.[21]

Newer Therapies

There have been several important recent advances in endoscopic hemostasis therapy. These are covered more extensively in other articles within this issue; however,

Table 2			
Some available clips and their features			
Clip	**Company**	**Opening Width**	**Special Features**
Resolution	Boston Scientific	11 mm	Reopens
Resolution 360	Boston Scientific	11 mm	Reopens and 360° rotation
QuickClip2	Olympus	7.5 mm	Rotatable
QuickClip2 Long	Olympus	9 mm	Rotatable
QuickClip Pro	Olympus	11 mm	Reopens and 360° rotation
Instinct Endoscopic Hemoclip	Cook Medical	16 mm	Reopens and 360° rotation
Clipmaster	Medwork	12 mm	360° rotation
Clipmaster3	Medwork	12 mm	360° rotation and deploys 3 consecutive clips
Viper Hemoclip	Diagmed Healthcare	11 mm	Reopens and rotatable

some are worth a brief mention here as their use is becoming commonplace in many centers.

Topically applied hemostatic powders or gels are being more widely used in peptic ulcer bleeding. Hemospray (Cook Medical) was the first of these agents to be licensed in Europe; however, is not yet cleared for use in the United States.[23] Hemospray is an inorganic hemostatic powder that is approved for use in nonvariceal upper GI bleeding. It is propelled by a carbon dioxide pressurized plastic catheter that is fed through the endoscope and sprayed at a distance of 1 to 2 cm from the bleeding site until the area is coated with powder. When the powder comes into contact with a bleeding site, it forms a confluent barrier and promotes thrombus formation.

Initial data on Hemospray as monotherapy in nonvariceal upper GI bleeding reported initial hemostasis rates of 85% to 95% and rebleeding rates of 10% to 15%.[23,24] Sinha and colleagues[25] recently reported on 20 patients to assess Hemospray use as a second agent combined with epinephrine injection, or as an adjunct to dual therapy with epinephrine and either clips or a thermal device. Initial hemostasis rate was 95% and overall rebleeding rate 16% (9% when used as an adjunct to conventional therapies). However, to date there are no randomized studies comparing hemostatic powders with standard endoscopic techniques for controlling upper GI bleeding. Further data on Hemostatic powders and other new techniques including the over the scope clip system and use of Doppler probes is discussed in detail in other articles.

MONOTHERAPY VERSUS COMBINATION THERAPY
Monotherapy

In the context of so many modalities available for the management of peptic ulcer bleeding, there have been many studies and metaanalyses aiming to identify the optimum therapeutic approach. As outlined in the individual therapies section, it has been shown that endoscopic therapy with injectable sclerosants and glue, thermal therapies, and mechanical therapies are significantly better at preventing rebleeding than no endoscopic therapy at all.[6,9,26]

Several metaanalyses have sought to compare individual therapies to identify whether any singular modality is superior. Trials assessing the injection of epinephrine alone versus other monotherapies such as heater probe, bipolar electrocoagulation, APC, fibrin glue, sclerosant, or clips have shown that injection of epinephrine alone is inferior in preventing rebleeding.[6,26–28] When thermal therapy was compared with sclerosant therapy alone in 1 metaanalysis, there was no significant difference in primary hemostasis (relative risk, 1.27; 95% confidence interval, 0.93–1.75).[6] When comparing mechanical therapy with thermal therapy, 1 metaanalysis found that clips were significantly better at reducing rebleeding rates, but did not reduce surgery or mortality.[26] Another study compared mechanical with both thermal and sclerosant monotherapies and found no difference in rebleeding.[6]

Combination Therapy

The question of whether single modality therapy is adequate or if combination therapy is more effective has been the topic of multiple trials and metaanalyses. A Cochrane review in 2014 assessed 19 randomized trials incorporating 2033 patients and concluded that a second hemostatic modality significantly reduced the risk of rebleeding and emergency surgery compared with epinephrine alone[27] (**Fig. 1**). Mortality was also reduced, but did not reach statistical significance. Therefore, it was concluded that epinephrine should not be used as monotherapy, but only in combination with

Review: Epinephrine injection versus epinephrine injection and a second endoscopic method in high-risk bleeding ulcers
Comparison: 1 Epinephrine versus epinephrine and any second endoscopic method
Outcome: 3 Recurrent and persistent bleeding overall rates with or without second-look endoscopy

Study or subgroup	Combined therapy n/N	Epinephrine alone n/N	Risk Ratio M-H,Random,95% CI	Weight	Risk Ratio M-H,Random,95% CI
Lo 2006	3/52	15/53		4.2 %	0.20 [0.06, 0.66]
Grgov 2012	2/28	10/30		3.1 %	0.21 [0.05, 0.89]
Kubba 1996	3/70	14/70		4.1 %	0.21 [0.06, 0.71]
Villanueva 1996	2/42	7/37		2.9 %	0.25 [0.06, 1.14]
Garrido 2002	3/40	12/45		4.1 %	0.28 [0.09, 0.93]
Park 2004	3/45	10/45		4.0 %	0.30 [0.09, 1.02]
Lin 1999	4/32	12/32		5.1 %	0.33 [0.12, 0.92]
Lee 1997	4/30	10/30		4.9 %	0.40 [0.14, 1.14]
Lin 1993	5/32	12/32		5.8 %	0.42 [0.17, 1.05]
Chung 1997	15/136	28/134		9.2 %	0.53 [0.30, 0.94]
Loizou 1991	3/21	5/21		3.6 %	0.60 [0.16, 2.20]
Chung 1999	5/42	8/41		5.0 %	0.61 [0.22, 1.71]
Balanzo 1990	5/32	6/32		4.7 %	0.83 [0.28, 2.46]
Pescatore 2002	14/65	17/70		8.7 %	0.89 [0.48, 1.65]
Choudari 1994	7/52	8/55		5.7 %	0.93 [0.36, 2.37]
Chung 1993	21/98	22/98		9.9 %	0.95 [0.56, 1.62]
Sollano 1991	2/29	2/32		1.9 %	1.10 [0.17, 7.34]
Chung 1996	16/79	14/81		8.4 %	1.17 [0.61, 2.24]
Villanueva 1993	8/33	4/30		4.6 %	1.82 [0.61, 5.43]
Total (95% CI)	**958**	**968**		**100.0 %**	**0.57 [0.43, 0.76]**

Total events: 125 (Combined therapy), 216 (Epinephrine alone)
Heterogeneity: Tau² = 0.14; Chi² = 29.11, df = 18 (p = .05); I² =38%
Test for overall effect: Z = 3.85 (p = .0001)
Test for subgroup differences: Not applicable

0.05   0.2   1   5   20
Combined therapy   Epinephrine alone

Fig. 1. Cochrane systematic review of epinephrine plus another modality versus epinephrine alone, 2014. CI, confidence interval. (*From* Vergara M, Bennett C, Calvet X, et al. Epinephrine injection versus epinephrine injection and a second endoscopic method in high-risk bleeding ulcers. Cochrane Database Syst Rev 2014;10:CD005584; with permission.)

a second modality. This finding is consistent with reports from several other metaanalyses.[6,26,27]

In 2007, Marmo and colleagues[27] reported no significant difference in outcomes when combination therapy with epinephrine and a thermal device was used compared with a thermal modality alone. This finding suggested that thermal monotherapy may be acceptable and may be safer than combination therapy. However, Barkun and colleagues[26] compared epinephrine and thermal device versus thermal alone and found reduced rebleeding with combination therapy; therefore, thermal monotherapy is generally not recommended. Interestingly, both metaanalyses reported that monotherapy with clips was as effective as combination therapy with clips and epinephrine; therefore, it also seems to be acceptable to use clips as monotherapy.[26,27]

ADVERSE EVENTS OF ENDOSCOPIC THERAPY

After endoscopic therapy, adverse events including perforation and therapy-induced bleeding can occur. Although more common with endoscopic therapy than with medical therapy alone, the difference was not statistically significant in a metaanalysis (0.8% vs 0.1%).[6]

Perforation and bleeding have the potential to occur with any endoscopic hemostasis modality. Thermal therapy has a reported perforation rate of 1.8% to 3.0% and can precipitate bleeding in up to 5.0% of patients.[16] Injection therapy complications are usually related to the substance being injected. However, there can also be technical problems, such as failure of the needle to extend from the sheath or separation from the catheter.[16] Endoscopic injection of epinephrine can be associated with bleeding, cardiac arrhythmias, and hypertension.[6] Injection of sclerosants can induce bleeding or cause perforation as well as systemic effects, such as fever and bacteremia.[6,15] Sclerotherapy-induced GI wall necrosis and arterial thrombosis leading to infarction has also been reported.[27]

Mechanical therapy adverse events include malfunction of the clipping device leading to failure of the clip to separate from the catheter or premature deployment.[16] However, a metaanalysis found no episodes of induced bleeding or perforation in 373 patients treated with clips and epinephrine.[6] This was the therapy with the lowest adverse event rate when compared with epinephrine alone or combination therapy with epinephrine plus sclerosant or with epinephrine plus a thermal modality.

A metaanalysis of 20 studies comparing combination therapy (epinephrine injection plus injection or thermal or mechanical method) versus monotherapy (injection, thermal, or mechanical alone) reported adverse event rates of 3.3% and 3.5%, respectively.[27] This study also reported that rates of therapy-induced bleeding were similar when comparing mono versus combination therapy; however, perforation rates were significantly higher with combination therapy. The perforations were most common in patients who underwent epinephrine and thermal combination therapy. A larger more recent metaanalysis by Laine and McQuaid[6] analyzed 75 randomized trials and reported only a 0.5% overall pooled adverse event rate for all therapeutic modalities.

SECOND LOOK ENDOSCOPY

There has always been a role for early repeat endoscopy in selected situations, such as poor initial endoscopic visualization or clinical concern regarding suboptimal initial endotherapy. However, it has been suggested that a routine, scheduled repeat endoscopy after initial hemostasis (usually performed within the next 24 hours) may be of benefit in identifying patients with persisting high-risk endoscopic stigmata and allow for an early opportunity to provide further endotherapy. A metaanalysis assessed 8 randomized trials and found that routine second look endoscopy did not significantly improve patient outcomes.[13] The 2 trials within the metaanalysis that reported a positive outcome for routine second look endoscopy included particularly high-risk patients. Wong and colleagues[29] aimed to identify independent risk factors for treatment failure after the administration of epinephrine injection and thermocoagulation in bleeding peptic ulcers. They found that a hemoglobin level of less than 10 g/dL, ulcer size of 2 cm or greater, systolic blood pressure of less than 100 mm Hg, fresh blood in the stomach, and active bleeding at endoscopy were all significantly associated with failure of initial endotherapy. These factors may help clinicians to identify higher risk patients who may benefit from a second look endoscopy. A randomized study by Saeed and colleagues[30] assessed selective repeat endoscopy in patients who were deemed at high risk of rebleeding as identified by the Baylor bleeding score. They demonstrated reduced rebleeding after repeat endoscopy in this high-risk group. Therefore, routine second look endoscopy is not recommended in patients with peptic ulcer bleeding. However, second look endoscopy in selected high-risk patients may be beneficial.

SUMMARY

Bleeding from peptic ulcer disease is a common condition and is associated with significant morbidity and mortality. Upper endoscopy and endoscopic hemostasis therapy has played an increasingly important role in diagnosis and management. It has become more accessible and therapeutic technology has become more advanced, which has reduced rebleeding rates, need for surgery and mortality rates over time.

The Forrest classification of stigmata of recent hemorrhage in peptic ulcer bleeding remains useful despite being developed 4 decades ago and gives valuable information on prognosis, in addition to guiding management. Forrest Ia, Ib and IIa lesions are at high risk of ongoing or recurrent bleeding and require endoscopic intervention. The management of Forrest IIb lesions (ulcers with adherent clot) remains controversial, because ulcers with this stigma are associated with greatly variable outcomes. The recommended course of action is to attempt clot removal with vigorous washing, to try and more accurately classify the underlying lesion and to clarify if endoscopic therapy is required.

Forrest IIc and III lesions are at low risk of rebleeding and have low mortality rates and, therefore, do not require endoscopic therapy. Studies have shown that the interpretation of ulcer stigmata using the Forrest classification can vary widely, even among experienced experts. It has been suggested that the Forrest classification could be modified to include low-risk, increased-risk, and high-risk categories in a bid to improve interobserver agreement. Other factors that predict an adverse outcome include ulcer size of greater than 2 cm, visible vessel size of greater than 2 mm, and ulcer location on the posterior duodenal wall or lesser curvature of the stomach.

Various endoscopic methods to achieve hemostasis in peptic ulcer bleeding are available. Traditionally, bleeding ulcers have been injected with dilute epinephrine to exert both a tamponade and vasoconstrictive effect. Injection with sclerosants or adhesives has been shown to be effective; however, they can lead to localized tissue damage and are rarely used. Thermal electrocoagulation using bipolar modalities or

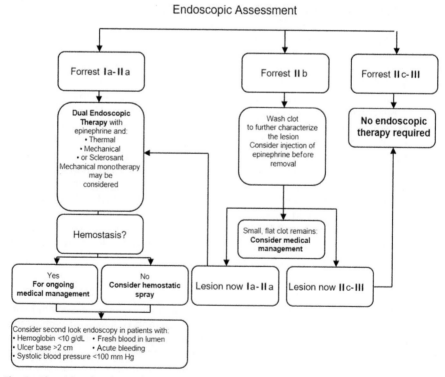

Fig. 2. Algorithm for the endoscopic management of peptic ulcer bleeding.

APC have been shown to be effective and relatively safe; however, there is a risk of perforation, particularly after prolonged application or repeated use. Mechanical therapy with through the scope clips is an effective and safe way to treat peptic ulcer bleeding and does not cause tissue injury.

Metaanalyses have been conducted to assess the efficacy of mono versus combination endoscopic therapy in the management of peptic ulcer bleeding. The results show that epinephrine should not be used as a single agent, but should be used in combination with a thermal or mechanical therapy. Evidence also suggests that clips are effective as monomodality therapy.

Recent advances in endoscopic hemostasis include new technologies such as hemostatic powders and over the scope clips. These modalities may be useful in situations where conventional methods fail or are difficult to apply and their use will be discussed in detail in subsequent articles.

Trials have assessed the merit of routine second look endoscopy after endoscopic therapy. A review of the evidence has not provided clear evidence that this approach improves outcome and, thus, it is not recommended routinely. However, second look endoscopy should be considered in patients felt to be at particularly high risk of ongoing or recurrent bleeding, or in those where initial endotherapy was deemed suboptimal. **Fig. 2** shows a suggested algorithm for endoscopic management of peptic ulcer bleeding.

REFERENCES

1. Gralnek IM, Dumonceau JM, Kuipers EJ, et al. Diagnosis and management of nonvariceal upper gastrointestinal hemorrhage: European Society of Gastrointestinal Endoscopy (ESGE) guideline. Endoscopy 2015;47:a1–46.
2. Laine L, Jensen DM. Management of patients with ulcer bleeding. Am J Gastroenterol 2012;107:345–60.
3. Hearnshaw SA, Logan RF, Lowe D, et al. Acute upper gastrointestinal bleeding in the UK: patient characteristics, diagnoses and outcomes in the 2007 UK audit. Gut 2011;60(10):1327–35.
4. Storey DW, Bown SG, Swain CP, et al. Endoscopic prediction of recurrent bleeding in peptic ulcers. N Engl J Med 1981;305:915–6.
5. Forrest JA, Finlayson ND, Shearman DJ. Endoscopy in gastrointestinal bleeding. Lancet 1974;2:394–7.
6. Laine L, McQuaid KR. Endoscopic therapy for bleeding ulcers: an evidence-based approach based on meta-analyses of randomized controlled trials. Clin Gastroenterol Hepatol 2009;7:33–47.
7. de Groot NL, van Oijen MG, Kessels K, et al. Reassessment of the predictive value of the Forrest classification for peptic ulcer rebleeding and mortality: can classification be simplified? Endoscopy 2014;46:46–52.
8. National Institute for Health and Care Excellence (NICE). 2016. Acute upper gastrointestinal bleeding in over 16s: management: NICE guideline (CG141).
9. Barkun AN, Bardou M, Kuipers EJ, et al. International consensus recommendations on the management of patients with nonvariceal upper gastrointestinal bleeding. Ann Intern Med 2010;152:101–13.
10. Waddell KM, Stanley AJ, Morris AJ. Endoscopy for upper gastrointestinal bleeding: where are we in 2017? Frontline Gastroenterol 2017;8:94–7.
11. Kahi CJ, Jensen DM, Sung JJ, et al. Endoscopic therapy versus medical therapy for bleeding peptic ulcer with adherent clot: a meta-analysis. Gastroenterology 2005;129:855–62.

12. Lau JY, Sung JJ, Chan AC, et al. Stigmata of hemorrhage in bleeding peptic ulcers: an interobserver agreement study among international experts. Gastrointest Endosc 1997;46:33–6.

13. El Ouali S, Barkun AN, Wyse J, et al. Is routine second-look endoscopy effective after endoscopic hemostasis in acute peptic ulcer bleeding? A meta-analysis. Gastrointest Endosc 2012;76:283–92.

14. Lin H, Hsieh H, Tseng, et al. A prospective, randomized trial or large- vs. small-volume injection of epinephrine for peptic ulcer bleeding. Gastrointest Endosc 2002;55:615–9.

15. Nunoue T, Takenaka R, Hori K, et al. A randomized trial of monopolar soft-mode coagulation versus heater probe thermocoagulation for peptic ulcer bleeding. J Clin Gastroenterol 2015;49:472–6.

16. Conway JD, Adler DG, Diehl DL, et al. Endoscopic hemostatic devices. Gastrointest Endosc 2009;69:987–96.

17. Ginsberg GG, Barkun AN, Bosco JJ, et al, American Society for Gastrointestinal Endoscopy. The argon plasma coagulator: February 2002. Gastrointest Endosc 2002;55:807–10.

18. Cipolletta L, Bianco MA, Rotondano G, et al. Prospective comparison of argon plasma coagulator and heater probe in the endoscopic treatment of major peptic ulcer bleeding. Gastrointest Endosc 1998;48:191–5.

19. Krejs GJ, Little KH, Westergaard H, et al. Laser photocoagulation for the treatment of acute peptic ulcer bleeding: a randomised controlled clinical trial. N Engl J Med 1987;316:1618–21.

20. Matthewson K, Swain CP, Bland M, et al. Randomized comparison of Nd YAG laser, heater probe, and no endoscopic therapy for bleeding peptic ulcers. Gastroenterology 1990;98:1239–44.

21. Raju GS, Gajula L. Endoclips for GI endoscopy. Gastrointest Endosc 2004;59:267–9.

22. Goelder SK, Brueckner J, Messmann H. Endoscopic hemostasis state of the art - nonvariceal bleeding. World J Gastrointest Endosc 2016;8:205–11.

23. Sung JJ, Luo D, Wu JC, et al. Early clinical experience of the safety and effectiveness of Hemospray in achieving hemostasis in patients with acute peptic ulcer bleeding. Endoscopy 2011;43:291–5.

24. Smith LA, Stanley AJ, Bergman JJ, et al. Hemospray application in nonvariceal upper gastrointestinal bleeding: results of the survey to evaluate the application of Hemospray in the luminal tract. J Clin Gastroenterol 2014;48:e89–92.

25. Sinha R, Lockman KA, Church NI, et al. The use of hemostatic spray as an adjunct to conventional hemostatic measures in high-risk non- variceal upper GI bleeding (with video). Gastrointest Endosc 2016;84:900–6.

26. Barkun AN, Martel M, Toubouti Y, et al. Endoscopic hemostasis in peptic ulcer bleeding for patients with high-risk lesions: a series of meta-analyses. Gastrointest Endosc 2009;69:786–99.

27. Marmo R, Rotondano G, Piscopo R, et al. Dual therapy versus monotherapy in the endoscopic treatment of high-risk bleeding ulcers: a meta-analysis of controlled trials. Am J Gastroenterol 2007;102:279–89.

28. Vergara M, Bennett C, Calvet X, et al. Epinephrine injection versus epinephrine injection and a second endoscopic method in high-risk bleeding ulcers. Cochrane Database Syst Rev 2014;(10):CD005584.

29. Wong SIC, Yu LM, Lau YH, et al. Prediction of therapeutic failure after epinephrine injection plus heater probe treatment in patients with bleeding peptic ulcer. Gut 2002;50:322–5.

30. Saeed ZA, Cole RA, Ramirez FC, et al. Endoscopic retreatment after successful initial hemostasis prevents ulcer rebleeding: a prospective randomized trial. Endoscopy 1996;28:288–94.

Endoscopic Management of Nonvariceal, Nonulcer Upper Gastrointestinal Bleeding

Michael A. Chang, MD*, Thomas J. Savides, MD

KEYWORDS

- Nonvariceal • Dieulafoy • Arteriovenous malformation • Mallory-Weiss tear
- Hemostasis • Malignant gastrointestinal bleeding • Topical spray hemostasis
- Over-the-scope clip

KEY POINTS

- Nonulcer acute upper gastrointestinal hemorrhage (UGIH) is a less common cause for UGIH compared with ulcer-related bleeding.
- The mainstay of endoscopic management of acute UGIH remains a combination of submucosal epinephrine injection with coaptive coagulation and/or hemostatic clips.
- A new modality of diagnosing nonulcer UGIH includes endoscopic Doppler probe identification of blood flow.
- Development of new modalities for the treatment of upper gastrointestinal hemorrhage has led to the introduction of topical sprays and over-the-scope clips.

INTRODUCTION

The most common cause for acute upper gastrointestinal hemorrhage (UGIH) is ulcer-related bleeding, which represents nearly 50% of all upper gastrointestinal (GI) bleeding. Nonulcer, nonvariceal bleeding is less common, representing approximately 25% to 35% of all upper GI bleeding.[1,2] The mortality associated with acute UGIH has been decreasing over the past 5 to 10 years with a study-reported mortality range of 2% to 5%. This figure is down from the 5% to 10% mortality observed previously.[1-5] This decrease may be attributable to the advent and increased use of proton pump inhibitor (PPI) medications, efforts to eradicate *Helicobacter pylori* infection, steady improvement in endoscopic equipment, including improvement in diagnostic imaging and available treatment modalities, and the shift to more restrictive blood transfusion strategies. Through the effective endoscopic management of acute UGIH, there is a

Disclosures: None.
Division of Gastroenterology, University of California, 9500 Gilman Drive #0956, La Jolla, CA 92093-0956, USA
* Corresponding author.
E-mail address: mac063@ucsd.edu

Gastrointest Endoscopy Clin N Am 28 (2018) 291–306
https://doi.org/10.1016/j.giec.2018.02.003
giendo.theclinics.com

reduction in the risk for recurrent bleeding, blood transfusion, need for surgery, and mortality.[6,7] The focus of this article is endoscopic therapy for nonvariceal, non-ulcer-related UGIH.

DIAGNOSIS

Determining if acute GI bleeding is from a source proximal to the ligament of Treitz can be aided by careful assessment of the clinical history, physical examination, and laboratory testing. Initial diagnosis of acute UGIH should focus on good history taking with an emphasis on clinical signs and symptoms related to GI bleeding. History of present illness should include timing of events, with focus on symptoms of blood volume loss (eg, presyncope, syncope, racing heart, chest pain). Specific questions should also include development of hematemesis or coffee grounds emesis, melena, or hematochezia. Alternative causes for the presence of GI blood should also be included, such as swallowed blood from large-volume epistaxis or oropharyngeal bleeding. Other focused questions should include surgical history, history of ulcer disease, history of liver disease or cirrhosis, history of gastroesophageal reflux disease, daily aspirin or nonsteroidal anti-inflammatory use, or chronic anticoagulation with medications, such as warfarin, oral direct thrombin inhibitors, or oral anti-Xa inhibitor medications. Assessing for high-risk clinical and examination features, such as melena, syncope, heart failure, liver disease, hypotension, and tachycardia, may be predictive of acute bleeding, which will likely need endoscopic intervention.[8]

Physical examination should initially focus on patient vital signs with special attention to hypotension, tachycardia, and orthostasis. Assessment for conjunctival pallor may indicate severe anemia, and assessment of the abdomen should include peritoneal signs, abdominal pain, and prior scars from previous surgeries. Careful assessment for stigmata of occult cirrhosis includes observation for scleral icterus, skin examination for spider angiomata on the chest, palmar erythema, jaundice, gynecomastia, ascites, firm shrunken liver, splenomegaly, and caput medusa. A problem-focused physical examination should also include a rectal examination for melena or hematochezia and possibly nasogastric lavage, which may aid in diagnosis of upper GI bleeding and in visualization at the time of endoscopy.[9]

Initial laboratory testing should include complete blood count, chemistry, and liver profile, biochemical, and coagulation studies. Blood testing may also include studies for type and cross-match in case transfusion is required. Special attention should be paid to the blood urea nitrogen level, the elevation of which is associated with increased need for endoscopic intervention and which may be elevated in acute upper GI bleeding because of small intestinal absorption of blood products.[8]

TREATMENT

Initial treatment is similar for all types of presumed acute UGIH and includes resuscitative efforts to correct hemodynamic instability with goal systolic blood pressure greater than 100 mm Hg and pulse rate less than 100 beats per minute. Patients should have intravenous (IV) access preferably via 2 large-bore peripheral IV catheters. If anemia is present, patients should undergo blood transfusion with goal hemoglobin greater than 7 g/dL, or possibly higher for patients with known ischemic cardiovascular disease or Childs class C cirrhosis.[1] Thrombocytopenia should be corrected with goal level greater than 50,000/mm^3 and prothrombin time less than 15 seconds.

Gastroenterology services should be requested by admitting physicians as soon as possible to expedite appropriate care and to determine timing of endoscopic interventions is needed. Initial medical therapy for presumed acute UGIH should include IV infusion of high-dose PPI medication, which reduces the need for endoscopic intervention.[10–12] Patients with suspicion of variceal bleeding should be considered for empiric IV octreotide infusion and treatment with antibiotics.[13,14]

After appropriate resuscitative efforts have been made, endoscopy can be pursued. Patients with ongoing active hemorrhage should be considered for admission into an intensive care unit, and endotracheal intubation should also be considered. Patients who are hemodynamically stable without evidence of ongoing bleeding should be considered for endoscopy on an urgent basis within 24 hours of hospital admission.[15]

The remainder of this article focuses on disease-specific causes of acute nonulcer, nonvariceal UGIH (**Box 1**).

ESOPHAGITIS

Patients with severe erosive esophagitis can present with hematemesis and melena (**Fig. 1**). Severe esophagitis is most commonly the result of untreated gastroesophageal reflux disease.[16] Other, rarer causes of severe esophagitis with bleeding complications include pill esophagitis, infections such as cytomegalovirus, herpes simplex virus, or candida.[17–19] Risk factors for bleeding esophagitis include moderate to severe esophagitis, cirrhosis, and concurrent anticoagulation therapy.[20] The gold standard in diagnosis of esophagitis is upper endoscopy. Endoscopic therapy generally has no role unless active focal bleeding is seen from an ulceration or an esophageal mucosal tear. Endoscopic treatment options include submucosal injection of 1:10,000 dilution epinephrine, hemoclip, and coaptive coagulation therapy (using a contact thermal probe). Hemostatic spray has been used on a limited number of patients with initial control of bleeding in 6 of 6 patients and recurrent bleeding on 1 of the 6 treated patients.[21] Generally, patients should be treated with once daily PPI and repeat endoscopy performed in 8 to 12 weeks to assess for healing and to rule out underlying Barrett's esophagus.

Box 1
Various causes for nonvariceal, nonulcer upper gastrointestinal bleeding

Esophagitis

Arterial aneurysm

Mallory-Weiss tear

Hemosuccus pancreaticus

Cameron lesions

Hemobilia

Dieulafoy

Aortoenteric fistula

Upper gastrointestinal malignancy

Anastomotic bleeding

Arteriovenous malformation

Acute esophageal necrosis

Telangiectasia

Atrial-esophageal fistula

Gastric antral vascular ectasia

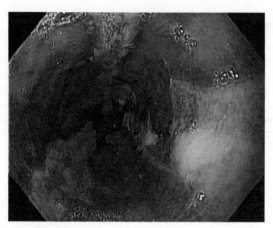

Fig. 1. Severe distal esophagitis.

MALLORY-WEISS TEARS

Mallory-Weiss tears are mucosal or submucosal lacerations that occur at or near the gastroesophageal junction and extend distally typically into a hernia or along the gastric cardia (**Fig. 2**). Patients generally present with hematemesis or coffee grounds emesis. Clinical history typically includes a history of multiple successive episodes of nonbloody emesis or retching followed by hematemesis; however, Mallory-Weiss tear may occur with a single retch or severe hiccups.[22,23] The cause of the tear is thought to emanate from a combination of increased intra-abdominal pressure in conjunction with a shearing force caused by additional negative intrathoracic pressure. Endoscopic evaluation should include forward (en face) and retroflexed views of the gastroesophageal junction because tears may not be readily visible on forward view. Mallory-Weiss tears may be actively spurting, oozing blood, or clean-based lesions. Active bleeding can be treated with a combination of submucosal epinephrine injection followed by through-the-scope clip or thermal coagulation therapy. The use of argon plasma coagulation (APC) has been described in the treatment of Mallory-Weiss tears and may be as effective as heater probe therapy.[24] Additional methods

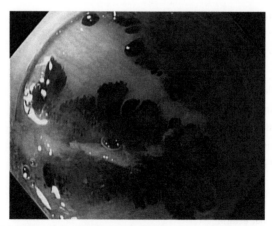

Fig. 2. Mallory-Weiss tear of the distal esophagus.

of achieving hemostasis include band ligation therapy, which was shown in consecutive patients to reduce the risk for rebleeding when compared with endoscopic clipping plus epinephrine injection.[25] In addition, over-the-scope clips and hemostatic spray have also been used to treat Mallory-Weiss tears and may be effective.[21,26,27]

CAMERON LESIONS

Cameron lesions are linear ulcerations or erosions within a hiatal hernia sac in the proximal stomach near the diaphragmatic pinch (**Fig. 3**).[28] Cameron lesions are caused by mechanical trauma and localized ischemia of the gastric mucosa as the stomach slides against the diaphragm in addition to acid peptic injury. Cameron lesions typically lead to chronic blood loss anemia but occasionally can result in massive acute upper GI bleeding.[29] Treatment of acute, focal bleeding from Cameron lesions includes submucosal injection of dilute epinephrine, thermal therapy, and endoscopic clipping. Medical therapy with PPI remains the treatment of choice, and surgical correction is an option for patients with refractory disease.

DIEULAFOY LESIONS

A Dieulafoy lesion is a non-ulcer-associated, large, submucosal artery that lies close to the mucosal surface and can result in massive acute GI bleeding (**Fig. 4**). These lesions account for 1% to 2% of all upper GI bleeding, are typically located in the gastric fundus, within 6 cm of the gastroesophageal junction, although lesions in the duodenum, small intestine, and colon have been reported.[30] The cause for these lesions is unknown; however, congenital and acquired causes may contribute to their development.

Dieulafoy lesions can often be missed during endoscopic evaluation due to their small size, the intermittent nature of bleeding, and the lack of surrounding stigmata, such as ulceration. When encountered, Dieulafoy lesions may be found to be spurting or with active oozing blood. Endoscopic Doppler ultrasound has been described in identification and treatment of these lesions.[31] Typical endoscopic therapies used to treat bleeding Dieulafoy lesions include submucosal injection therapy with epinephrine, coaptive bipolar coagulation, or mechanical therapy using clips. Placement of a submucosal tattoo (eg, India ink) at the site of the Dieulafoy lesions should be

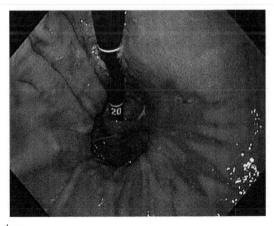

Fig. 3. Cameron ulcer.

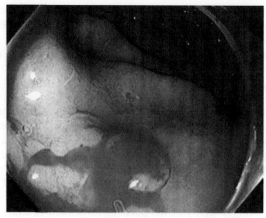

Fig. 4. Bleeding Dieulafoy lesion in the stomach.

considered in case rebleeding occurs and repeat treatment is needed. Additional endoscopic treatments that have been described include band ligation, over-the-scope clip, and ultrasound-guided injection of sclerosant.[32–34] Although ultrasound-guided injection of sclerosant has been reported, at this time this modality should be reserved for refractory disease and should be attempted only by an expert endoscopist. Endoscopic hemostasis is typically achieved in more than 90% of patients presenting with Dieulafoy lesions.[35] Rebleeding occurs approximately 8% of the time and is a predictor of increased mortality.

UPPER GASTROINTESTINAL MALIGNANCY

Malignancies account for only a small percentage of acute upper GI bleeding, with reports as low as 1% to 5% of all bleeding.[36] Bleeding typically occurs from large, ulcerated masses in the esophagus, stomach, or duodenum (**Fig. 5**). The most common upper GI tumors associated with upper GI bleeding, listed in descending order, include adenocarcinoma of the stomach and esophagus, mesenchymal (GI stromal tumors), and metastatic disease.[36] Typically, endoscopic hemostasis is ineffective

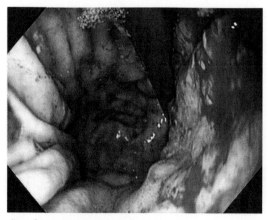

Fig. 5. Diffuse bleeding from a gastric cancer.

for diffuse tumor bleeding; however, for smaller lesions with active arterial bleeding or when high-risk stigmata are seen, these lesions can be treated with a combination of epinephrine injection, thermal coagulation, or clip. A relatively new endoscopic therapy is available to treat diffuse GI hemorrhage with the recent introduction of hemostatic powder/spray. This spray had been used in limited series with seemingly good results, implying immediate hemostasis in nearly 100% of cases and approximately 20% rebleeding risk.[37,38] A more recent series included more than 60 patients with tumor-related bleeding and reported greater than 95% immediate hemostasis, with 25% rebleeding rate at day 8 and 38% at day 30.[21] Given the high rate of rebleeding, surgical resection of the tumor should be considered when possible. When surgical resection is not an option, radiation therapy may be considered for hemostasis, with reports of greater than 70% effectiveness in achieving early hemostasis and rebleeding varying from 30% to 50%.[39,40]

ARTERIOVENOUS MALFORMATION

Arteriovenous malformations (AVM) are abnormal, congenital lesions, with direct connection between arterioles and venules, which bypass the normal capillary structure. The AVMs can occur anywhere in the GI tract, and bleeding lesions are typically flat red lesions and located within the submucosa. Rarely, these lesions may be polyploid and involve the full thickness of the GI wall, and their involvement may be extensive and include other organs such as the pancreas.[41] Other types of angiodysplasia are more common than AVM, and true AVMs are rare, accounting for approximately 1% of all acute upper GI bleeding.[42] Focal GI bleeding from small AVMs can be treated endoscopically with multimodality therapy, including epinephrine injection, thermal therapy, and endoscopic clips. However, given the nature of these lesions, further imaging with endoscopic ultrasound, computed tomography (CT), or angiography should be considered to rule out a more extensive lesion involvement, which may require angiographic embolization or surgical resection.[43]

TELANGIECTASIA

Telangiectasias are typically flat, red, spiderlike, small, isolated, dilated blood vessels within the mucosal and submucosal layers of the GI tract (**Fig. 6**). These lesions may

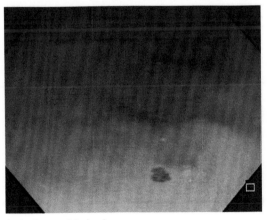

Fig. 6. Telangiectasia in the gastric body.

occur anywhere within the GI tract and are commonly found in the small bowel and colon. These lesions are commonly associated with hereditary hemorrhagic telangiectasia, left ventricular assist devices (LVAD), and aortic stenosis (Heyde syndrome). A recent review suggested that continuous flow LVAD bleeding most commonly occurs from angioectasias and carries a GI bleeding risk of 61% with rebleeding risk of up to 72%. This elevated bleeding risk is thought to occur through acquired von Willebrand factor deficiency and use of anticoagulation medications.[44] Bleeding may present as hematemesis, melena, hematochezia, or occult iron deficiency. Diagnosis typically consists of endoscopy and capsule enteroscopy when appropriate. When bleeding lesions are found, endoscopic treatment modalities include mechanical clip or thermal therapies, such as bipolar probe coagulation or APC.

GASTRIC ANTRAL VASCULAR ECTASIA

Gastric antral vascular ectasia (GAVE), also sometimes referred to as "watermelon stomach," appears as longitudinal rows of ectatic mucosal blood vessels that emanate from the pylorus and extend proximally into the antrum (**Fig. 7**). The underlying mechanism for the development of GAVE is unknown; however, GAVE is commonly associated with end-stage renal disease, scleroderma, and cirrhosis.[45] GAVE associated with cirrhosis may lack the typical appearance of "watermelon stomach" and have a more diffuse antral appearance. Patients typically present with iron deficiency anemia but may present with hematemesis or melena. Diagnosis is made by upper endoscopy. GAVE is commonly treated with thermal ablation therapy, such as APC, but bipolar coagulation and laser therapy are also used.[46] Typically, treatment to ablation requires multiple endoscopic treatment sessions 4 to 8 weeks apart to allow for interval healing. Repeated therapy has been shown to decrease the need for blood transfusion and hospitalization.[45] For refractory cases, cryoablation, band ligation, and radiofrequency ablation have been reported with success.[47–49]

ARTERIAL ANEURYSM

Visceral arterial aneurysms are rare, occurring in only 0.2% of the population, and are a rare cause for acute upper GI bleeding.[50] However, given the size of the vessels involved and high pressures, bleeding from arterial aneurysm is a life-threatening

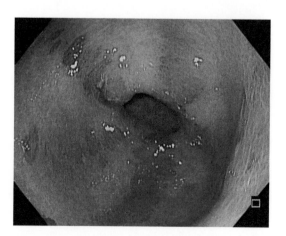

Fig. 7. GAVE.

emergency and carries a high mortality. Visceral artery aneurysms can be found in the hepatic artery, gastroduodenal artery, gastric arteries, splenic artery, and more rarely, superior and inferior mesenteric arteries. Aneurysmal dilation may occur from iatrogenic vascular trauma, congenital malformation, arteriosclerosis, or acute inflammation from pancreatitis. On endoscopy, lesions may appear as small or large, bulging, or polypoid lesions with stigmata of recent bleeding (**Fig. 8**). If aneurysm is suspected, then the preferred treatment is endovascular embolization or surgical repair.[51] Endoscopic treatment should be avoided given the high risk for the development of uncontrollable bleeding; however, treatment with over-the-scope clipping has been reported.[52,53]

HEMOSUCCUS PANCREATICUS

Hemosuccus pancreaticus is a rare cause for upper GI bleeding that occurs most in patients with a history of acute pancreatitis, chronic pancreatitis, pancreatic pseudocyst, pancreatic cancer, as a result of pancreatic duct manipulation following endoscopic retrograde cholangiopancreatography (ERCP), or secondary to rupture of a splenic arty aneurysm into the pancreatic duct.[54] Hemosuccus pancreaticus should be considered in patients with prior pancreatitis who present with acute upper GI bleeding. Diagnosis can be made endoscopically using a side-viewing endoscope (duodenoscope) or a forward-viewing endoscope with distal attachment cap, provided that the ampullary orifice can be visualized. Management is usually via endovascular embolization or less commonly with surgical resection.

HEMOBILIA

Hemobilia may occur because of complications related to hepatocellular carcinoma, hepatic AVM, hepatic artery aneurysm, parasitic infection, or as a complication from liver biopsy, percutaneous transhepatic cholangiography, transjugular intrahepatic portosystemic shunt, or following ERCP (**Fig. 9**). Patients may present with a combination of overt GI bleeding and elevated liver biochemical tests, suggesting biliary obstruction. Hemobilia should be suspected in a patient with prior pancreatitis or recent biliary manipulation. If the clinical suspicion is high, then CT imaging with

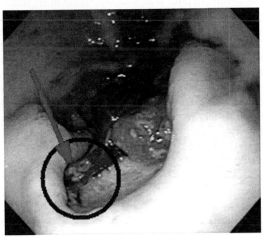

Fig. 8. Arterial aneurysm (*circle and arrow*) seen at the base of a gastric ulcer.

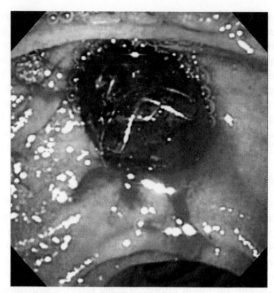

Fig. 9. Hemobilia seen within a metal biliary stent.

contrast or MRI imaging can be pursued. The diagnosis can be confirmed using a side-viewing endoscope or a forward-viewing endoscope with distal attachment cap, provided that the ampullary orifice can be visualized. Treatment is typically with endovascular embolization, or rarely, surgery. Endoscopic treatments are limited given the location of bleeding; however, if bleeding has been controlled and biliary obstruction is present, then biliary stenting may be considered.

AORTOENTERIC FISTULA

Aortoenteric (AE) fistula is a rare, but dreaded cause of acute upper GI bleeding that usually presents with acute, massive hemorrhage and carries with it with a high mortality.[55] The fistulization of the aorta to the GI tract can develop from chronic inflammation from infection or otherwise related to prior endovascular repair of an abdominal aortic aneurysm, or it may develop de novo in the absence of prior vascular manipulation. De novo fistulas typically occur in the duodenum, whereas endovascular fistulas commonly occur in the jejunum or ileum. Bleeding may present as massive life-threatening bleeding or the so-called herald bleed, whereby massive hemorrhage occurs and then spontaneously resolves. If a patient with prior aortic aneurysm or aortic aneurysmal repair presents with massive GI hemorrhage, then CT imaging should be pursued, preferably before endoscopy in order to expedite the diagnosis of a potentially life-threatening bleed and to avoid misidentification and attempted endoscopic treatment of an AE fistula at the time of endoscopy. Endoscopy may identify the cause of bleeding; however, it will be normal in more than 50% of patients with AE fistula.[56] Attempt at endoscopic treatment should be strictly avoided, and emergent consultation with vascular surgery should be initiated, because surgical removal of the graft is the treatment of choice.

ANASTOMOTIC BLEEDING

Bleeding from surgical GI anastomosis is a relatively rare complication and is reported to occur in approximately 4% of patients following bariatric surgery after 8 years of clinical follow-up (**Fig. 10**).[57] The cause of anastomotic bleeding emanates from local ischemia and the subsequent formation of erosions or ulcerations and bleeding. Anastomotic bleeding may be diffuse or focal due to ulceration. Bleeding can be treated with a combination of submucosal epinephrine injection, clipping, and/or thermal coagulation. Also, over-the-scope clips and hemostatic spray have been described to control anastomotic bleeding.[58,59]

ACUTE ESOPHAGEAL NECROSIS: "BLACK ESOPHAGUS"

Rarely, acute upper GI bleeding may occur as a result of an ischemic event. Acute esophageal necrosis (AEN), also commonly referred to a "black esophagus," can occur as a result of localized ischemia to the esophageal mucosa. AEN may involve the entire esophagus, but typically involves the distal third of the esophagus and abruptly ends at the gastroesophageal junction (**Fig. 11**). AEN typically presents with hematemesis and melena in up to 70% of cases and carries a high mortality of more than 30%.[60] The exact mechanism of ischemia is unknown; however, most likely there is an underlying deficit in blood flow to the esophagus (eg, hypotension, atherosclerosis) followed by a secondary insult, such as acid reflux or recurrent vomiting, which further reduces mucosal blood flow. The diagnostic test of choice is endoscopy. When bleeding is encountered, it is typically diffuse oozing and does not require endoscopic intervention. The treatment of choice is medical management with PPI medication, supportive care, surgical consultation, and close monitoring for clinical deterioration, which may indicate that esophageal perforation has occurred.

ATRIAL ESOPHAGEAL FISTULA

Another very uncommon cause for acute upper GI bleeding is the formation of an atrial esophageal fistula. Atrial esophageal fistula typically occurs as an adverse event from cardiac catheter ablation of atrial fibrillation. This event is an exceedingly rare adverse event, occurring in approximately 0.25% to less than 0.1% of all ablation procedures.[61] The cause of such an adverse event is due to the left atrial proximity to the esophagus within the mediastinum, which, under the correct circumstances, can lead to direct thermal injury of the esophagus and the end

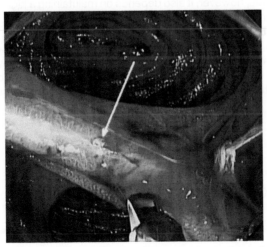

Fig. 10. Previously actively bleeding visible vessel (*arrow*) seen at a jejunojejunal anastomosis.

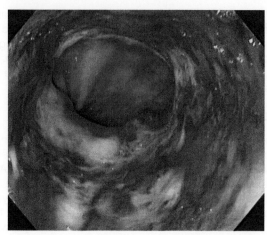

Fig. 11. AEN in the distal esophagus. Note the sparing of the gastric mucosa.

arterioles leading to focal ischemia, ulceration, and fistula formation. Fistula formation and bleeding are typically delayed, occurring 1 to 6 weeks after the ablation procedure. When the fistula forms, it typically forms a one-way valve from the esophagus into the left atrium, which commonly presents with embolic stroke in more than half of patients. If atrial esophageal fistula is suspected, then the diagnostic test of choice is CT imaging, because endoscopy performed with positive pressure insufflation may precipitate an embolic stroke. Although endoscopic management has been described in a single case report with fistula closure, early surgical repair is likely the treatment of choice because the mortality may approach 100% without surgical treatment.[62]

SUMMARY

Although less common than peptic ulcer disease and variceal bleeding, nonvariceal nonulcer acute UGIH is a frequent cause for acute upper GI bleeding. Diagnosis is typically endoscopic; however, it also depends on maintaining a high clinical suspicion for the less common causes, such as hemobilia, hemosuccus pancreaticus, arterial aneurysm, and AE fistula. Treatment options vary widely depending on the cause of bleeding, but the mainstay of endoscopic therapy remains submucosal epinephrine injection in combination with endoscopic clipping or thermal therapy. With the introduction of novel devices such as the over-the-scope clips and hemostatic spray, the ability to control acute upper GI bleeding without the need for surgery continues to improve.

REFERENCES

1. Villanueva C, Colomo A, Bosch A, et al. Transfusion strategies for acute upper gastrointestinal bleeding. N Engl J Med 2013;368(1):11–21.
2. Lau JY, Leung WK, Wu JC, et al. Omeprazole before endoscopy in patients with gastrointestinal bleeding. N Engl J Med 2007;356(16):1631–40.
3. Jairath V, Kahan BC, Gray A, et al. Restrictive versus liberal blood transfusion for acute upper gastrointestinal bleeding (TRIGGER): a pragmatic, open-label, cluster randomised feasibility trial. Lancet 2015;386(9989):137–44.

4. Sung JJ, Barkun A, Kuipers EJ, et al. Intravenous esomeprazole for prevention of recurrent peptic ulcer bleeding: a randomized trial. Ann Intern Med 2009;150(7): 455–64.
5. Hussain H, Lapin S, Cappell MS. Clinical scoring systems for determining the prognosis of gastrointestinal bleeding. Gastroenterol Clin North Am 2000;29(2): 445–64.
6. Han YJ, Cha JM, Park JH, et al. Successful endoscopic hemostasis is a protective factor for rebleeding and mortality in patients with nonvariceal upper gastrointestinal bleeding. Dig Dis Sci 2016;61(7):2011–8.
7. Jensen DM, Kovacs TO, Jutabha R, et al. Randomized trial of medical or endoscopic therapy to prevent recurrent ulcer hemorrhage in patients with adherent clots. Gastroenterology 2002;123(2):407–13.
8. Blatchford O, Murray WR, Blatchford M. A risk score to predict need for treatment for upper-gastrointestinal haemorrhage. Lancet 2000;356(9238):1318–21.
9. Lee SD, Kearney DJ. A randomized controlled trial of gastric lavage prior to endoscopy for acute upper gastrointestinal bleeding. J Clin Gastroenterol 2004;38(10):861–5.
10. Enns RA, Gagnon YM, Rioux KP, et al. Cost-effectiveness in Canada of intravenous proton pump inhibitors for all patients presenting with acute upper gastrointestinal bleeding. Aliment Pharmacol Ther 2003;17(2):225–33.
11. Al-Sabah S, Barkun AN, Herba K, et al. Cost-effectiveness of proton-pump inhibition before endoscopy in upper gastrointestinal bleeding. Clin Gastroenterol Hepatol 2008;6(4):418–25.
12. Dorward S, Sreedharan A, Leontiadis GI, et al. Proton pump inhibitor treatment initiated prior to endoscopic diagnosis in upper gastrointestinal bleeding. Cochrane Database Syst Rev 2006;(4):CD005415.
13. Fernandez J, Ruiz del Arbol L, Gómez C, et al. Norfloxacin vs ceftriaxone in the prophylaxis of infections in patients with advanced cirrhosis and hemorrhage. Gastroenterology 2006;131(4):1049–56 [quiz: 1285].
14. Corley DA, Cello JP, Adkisson W, et al. Octreotide for acute esophageal variceal bleeding: a meta-analysis. Gastroenterology 2001;120(4):946–54.
15. Spiegel BM, Vakil NB, Ofman JJ. Endoscopy for acute nonvariceal upper gastrointestinal tract hemorrhage: is sooner better? A systematic review. Arch Intern Med 2001;161(11):1393–404.
16. Moayyedi P, Talley NJ. Gastro-oesophageal reflux disease. Lancet 2006; 367(9528):2086–100.
17. Kumar A. Massive upper gastrointestinal bleeding due to Candida esophagitis. South Med J 1994;87(6):669–71.
18. Smith LA, Gangopadhyay M, Gaya DR. Catastrophic gastrointestinal complication of systemic immunosuppression. World J Gastroenterol 2015;21(8):2542–5.
19. Canalejo Castrillero E, García Durán F, Cabello N, et al. Herpes esophagitis in healthy adults and adolescents: report of 3 cases and review of the literature. Medicine (Baltimore) 2010;89(4):204–10.
20. Costa ND, Cadiot G, Merle C, et al. Bleeding reflux esophagitis: a prospective 1-year study in a university hospital. Am J Gastroenterol 2001;96(1):47–51.
21. Haddara S, Jacques J, Lecleire S, et al. A novel hemostatic powder for upper gastrointestinal bleeding: a multicenter study (the "GRAPHE" registry). Endoscopy 2016;48(12):1084–95.
22. Dwivedi S, Al-Hamid H, Warren BJ. Mallory-Weiss tear after violent hiccups: a rare association. J Community Hosp Intern Med Perspect 2017;7(1):37–9.

23. Brown JD. Hiccups: an unappreciated cause of the mallory-weiss syndrome. Am J Med 2015;128(12):e19–20.

24. Akin M, Alkan E, Tuna Y, et al. Comparison of heater probe coagulation and argon plasma coagulation in the management of Mallory-Weiss tears and high-risk ulcer bleeding. Arab J Gastroenterol 2017;18(1):35–8.

25. Lecleire S, Antonietti M, Iwanicki-Caron I, et al. Endoscopic band ligation could decrease recurrent bleeding in Mallory-Weiss syndrome as compared to haemostasis by hemoclips plus epinephrine. Aliment Pharmacol Ther 2009;30(4): 399–405.

26. Skinner M, Gutierrez JP, Neumann H, et al. Over-the-scope clip placement is effective rescue therapy for severe acute upper gastrointestinal bleeding. Endosc Int Open 2014;2(1):E37–40.

27. Giles H, Lal D, Gerred S, et al. Efficacy and safety of TC-325 (HemosprayTM) for non-variceal upper gastrointestinal bleeding at Middlemore Hospital: the early New Zealand experience. N Z Med J 2016;129(1446):38–43.

28. Cameron AJ, Higgins JA. Linear gastric erosion. A lesion associated with large diaphragmatic hernia and chronic blood loss anemia. Gastroenterology 1986; 91(2):338–42.

29. Kapadia S, Jagroop S, Kumar A. Cameron ulcers: an atypical source for a massive upper gastrointestinal bleed. World J Gastroenterol 2012;18(35): 4959–61.

30. Jeon HK, Kim GH. Endoscopic management of Dieulafoy's lesion. Clin Endosc 2015;48(2):112–20.

31. Jaspersen D. Dieulafoy's disease controlled by Doppler ultrasound endoscopic treatment. Gut 1993;34(6):857–8.

32. Folvik G, Nesje LB, Berstad A, et al. Endosonography-guided endoscopic band ligation of Dieulafoy's malformation: a case report. Endoscopy 2001;33(7):636–8.

33. García de la Filia I, Hernanz N, Vázquez Sequeiros E, et al. Recurrent gastrointestinal bleeding secondary to Dieulafoy's lesion successfully treated with endoscopic ultrasound-guided sclerosis. Gastroenterol Hepatol 2017. [Epub ahead of print].

34. Gomez V, Kyanam Kabir Baig KR, Lukens FJ, et al. Novel treatment of a gastric Dieulafoy lesion with an over-the-scope clip. Endoscopy 2013;45(Suppl 2 UCTN):E71.

35. Park SH, Lee DH, Park CH, et al. Predictors of rebleeding in upper gastrointestinal Dieulafoy lesions. Clin Endosc 2015;48(5):385–91.

36. Savides TJ, Jensen DM, Cohen J, et al. Severe upper gastrointestinal tumor bleeding: endoscopic findings, treatment, and outcome. Endoscopy 1996; 28(2):244–8.

37. Chen YI, Barkun AN, Soulellis C, et al. Use of the endoscopically applied hemostatic powder TC-325 in cancer-related upper GI hemorrhage: preliminary experience (with video). Gastrointest Endosc 2012;75(6):1278–81.

38. Leblanc S, Vienne A, Dhooge M, et al. Early experience with a novel hemostatic powder used to treat upper GI bleeding related to malignancies or after therapeutic interventions (with videos). Gastrointest Endosc 2013;78(1):169–75.

39. Kondoh C, Shitara K, Nomura M, et al. Efficacy of palliative radiotherapy for gastric bleeding in patients with unresectable advanced gastric cancer: a retrospective cohort study. BMC Palliat Care 2015;14:37.

40. Asakura H, Hashimoto T, Harada H, et al. Palliative radiotherapy for bleeding from advanced gastric cancer: is a schedule of 30 Gy in 10 fractions adequate? J Cancer Res Clin Oncol 2011;137(1):125–30.

41. Uchida E, Aimoto T, Nakamura Y, et al. Pancreatic arteriovenous malformation involving adjacent duodenum with gastrointestinal bleeding: report of a case. J Nippon Med Sch 2006;73(6):346–50.

42. Loperfido S, Baldo V, Piovesana E, et al. Changing trends in acute upper-GI bleeding: a population-based study. Gastrointest Endosc 2009;70(2):212–24.

43. Ng SC, Thomas-Gibson S, Harbin LJ, et al. Gastric arteriovenous malformation: a rare cause of upper GI bleed. Gastrointest Endosc 2009;69(1):155–6 [discussion: 156].

44. Cushing K, Kushnir V. Gastrointestinal bleeding following LVAD placement from top to bottom. Dig Dis Sci 2016;61(6):1440–7.

45. Dulai GS, Jensen DM, Kovacs TO, et al. Endoscopic treatment outcomes in watermelon stomach patients with and without portal hypertension. Endoscopy 2004;36(1):68–72.

46. Ng I, Lai KC, Ng M. Clinical and histological features of gastric antral vascular ectasia: successful treatment with endoscopic laser therapy. J Gastroenterol Hepatol 1996;11(3):270–4.

47. Trindade AJ, Inamdar S, Sejpal DV. Nitrous oxide CryoBalloon therapy of refractory gastric antral vascular ectasia. Endoscopy 2017;49(9):923–4.

48. Zepeda-Gómez S, Sultanian R, Teshima C, et al. Gastric antral vascular ectasia: a prospective study of treatment with endoscopic band ligation. Endoscopy 2015; 47(6):538–40.

49. Dray X, Repici A, Gonzalez P, et al. Radiofrequency ablation for the treatment of gastric antral vascular ectasia. Endoscopy 2014;46(11):963–9.

50. Haruta N, Asahara T, Fukuda T, et al. Ruptured superior mesenteric artery aneurysm occurring in association with a heterotopic pancreas: report of a case. Surg Today 1999;29(7):656–9.

51. Cordova AC, Sumpio BE. Visceral artery aneurysms and pseudoaneurysms—should they all be managed by endovascular techniques? Ann Vasc Dis 2013; 6(4):687–93.

52. El Douaihy Y, Kesavan M, Deeb L, et al. Over-the-scope clip to the rescue of a bleeding gastroduodenal artery pseudoaneurysm. Gastrointest Endosc 2016; 84(5):854–5.

53. Nishiyama N, Mori H, Kobara H, et al. Endoscopic management with over-the-scope clips for intestinal bleeding of Behcet's disease. Gastrointest Endosc 2015;81(5):1275–6.

54. Han B, Song ZF, Sun B. Hemosuccus pancreaticus: a rare cause of gastrointestinal bleeding. Hepatobiliary Pancreat Dis Int 2012;11(5):479–88.

55. Busuttil SJ, Goldstone J. Diagnosis and management of aortoenteric fistulas. Semin Vasc Surg 2001;14(4):302–11.

56. Deijen CL, Tsai A, Koedam TW, et al. Clinical outcomes and case volume effect of transanal total mesorectal excision for rectal cancer: a systematic review. Tech Coloproctol 2016;20(12):811–24.

57. Fernandez-Esparrach G, Córdova H, Bordas JM, et al. Endoscopic management of the complications of bariatric surgery. Experience of more than 400 interventions. Gastroenterol Hepatol 2011;34(3):131–6 [in Spanish].

58. Parsi MA, Jang S. Hemospray for diffuse anastomotic bleeding. Gastrointest Endosc 2014;80(6):1170.

59. Tontini GE, Naegel A, Albrecht H, et al. Successful over-the-scope clip (OTSC) treatment for severe bleeding due to anastomotic dehiscence. Endoscopy 2013;45(Suppl 2 UCTN):E343–4.

60. Gurvits GE, Shapsis A, Lau N, et al. Acute esophageal necrosis: a rare syndrome. J Gastroenterol 2007;42(1):29–38.
61. Kapur S, Barbhaiya C, Deneke T, et al. Esophageal injury and atrioesophageal fistula caused by ablation for atrial fibrillation. Circulation 2017;136(13):1247–55.
62. Shiraishi M, Morita H, Muramatsu K, et al. Successful non-operative management of left atrioesophageal fistula following catheter ablation. Surg Today 2014;44(8): 1565–8.

Emerging Endoscopic Treatments for Nonvariceal Upper Gastrointestinal Hemorrhage

Alvaro Martínez-Alcalá, MD[a], Klaus Mönkemüller, MD, PhD[b],*

KEYWORDS

- Nonvariceal upper gastrointestinal bleeding • Over-the-scope clip • Ovesco
- Hemospray • Radiofrequency ablation • Cryotherapy • Endoscopic suturing devices
- Cellulose

KEY POINTS

- There is a large number of emerging devices for treating nonvariceal upper gastrointestinal hemorrhage.
- Most devices will never enter clinical practice.
- The few devices that have proven efficacy and effectiveness are the over-the-scope clip and hemostatic sprays, both of which are currently being used routinely in many endoscopic units.

INTRODUCTION

Upper gastrointestinal (GI) hemorrhage (UGIH) remains a common clinical problem caused by a broad spectrum of etiologic factors (**Table 1**). Although this article focuses on emerging endoscopic therapies for dealing with nonvariceal UGIH (NVUGIH), it emphasizes that whenever treating a patient with UGIH a structured approach should be followed.[1–3] The classic ABCDE approach is still current, in which A stands for airways (securing and protecting), B for breathing (eg, supplying oxygen, consider mechanical ventilation), C for circulation (placement of 2 large-bore intravenous lines and resuscitation with intravenous crystalloids and, if necessary, blood and plasma), D for drugs (eg, use of erythromycin to clear clots from the stomach, intravenous proton pump inhibitors for peptic ulcer bleeding, vasoactive medications; eg, terlipressin or

Disclosure Statement: K. Mönkemüller has been speaker and consultant for Cook Medical, USA, and Ovesco, Germany.
[a] Department of Gastroenterology, Hospital Universitario Infanta Leonor, Madrid, Spain;
[b] Department of Visceral Surgery, Division of Endoscopy, Frankenwaldklinik, Kronach, Germany
* Corresponding author.
E-mail address: moenkemueller@yahoo.com

Table 1
Important causes of upper gastrointestinal hemorrhage

Variceal bleeding	Esophageal varices	Portal hypertension or hepatic disease
	Gastric varices	Hepatic disease or prehepatic thrombosis
Nonvariceal bleeding	Peptic ulcer disease	Stomach and gastric ulcers, induced by *Helicobacter pylori* and nonsteroidal antiinflammatory drugs
	Erosive esophagitis	
	Gastric antral vascular ectasias	
	Erosive gastritis and/or duodenitis	
	Anastomotic ulcers	
Neoplastic lesions	Tumors of the oropharynx, esophagus, and stomach	Cancer, lipomas, gastrointestinal stromal tumors
Vascular malformations	Dieulafoy lesions	
	Angiodysplasias	
	Hemophilia, aortoenteric fistula	
Others	Mallory-Weiss lesions	
	Cameron ulcers	
Iatrogenic lesions	Postendoscopic resection (endoscopic mucosal resection or endoscopic submucosal dissection)	

octreotide for variceal bleeding), and E for endoscopy (used for diagnostic; ie, risk stratification, and therapeutic purposes). Unfortunately, it is very common for treating physicians to call in the endoscopy team before any of the initial critical steps of the ABCD have been accomplished. When the endoscopist receives the call, the ABCD should have been accomplished so that endoscopy can proceed in a properly monitored and hemodynamically resuscitated patient, either in the emergency room, intermediate care, or intensive care unit.[1]

Despite major improvements in endoscopic devices and therapeutic endoscopy, rebleeding rates and mortality have remained the same for several decades.[1-5] Often, rebleeding occurs in ulcers with a visible vessel and complex or large fibrotic lesions (**Figs. 1** and **2**). Therefore, much interest has been paid to emerging therapeutic devices, such as the over-the-scope clip (OTSC) and hemostatic sprays[6-30] (**Fig. 3**). Other emerging technologies, such as radiofrequency ablation (RFA), endoscopic suturing devices, ultrasound-guided angiotherapy, and oxidized cellulose, are also being investigated to improve therapeutic outcomes in specific situations[30-47] (**Fig. 4**). **Table 2** summarizes the most important emerging endoscopic devices currently in clinical use.[6-48]

OVER-THE-SCOPE CLIP

The OTSC (Ovesco, Tübingen, Germany), which is also referred to as the bear claw, is an endoscopic clipping device designed for tissue approximation.[6-8] The device, which is made of nitinol, was originally used for the closure of fistulae and endoscopic perforations.[6,9] However, its uses have been expanded to include therapy for bleeding lesions, resection of submucosal tumors, and even esophageal stent fixation.[6-10] Currently, a main use is the treatment of NVUGIH[11,12] (see **Figs. 2–4**; **Fig. 5**). Indeed, the OTSC device may become a better device to treat bleeding ulcers located in

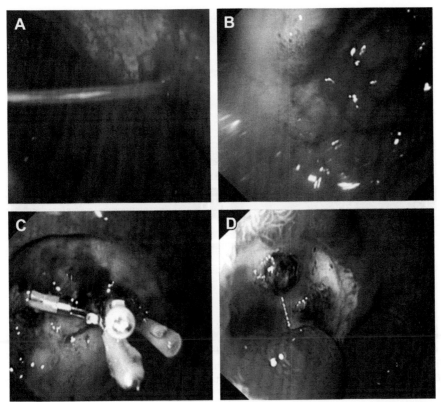

Fig. 1. Complex lesions causing NVUGIH. (*A*) Spurting vessel. (*B*) Fibrotic ulcer with bleeding vessel. (*C*) Multiple clips are often necessary to induce hemostasis. (*D*) Large, fibrotic ulcer with visible vessel. The ulcer is located posteriorly, making endoscopic application of therapy difficult because the working channel of most gastroscopes is on the left side.

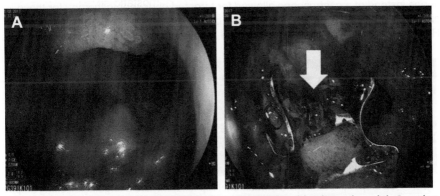

Fig. 2. Over-the-scope clip (OTSC) application on complex, bleeding ulcer. (*A*) Complex, fibrotic, bleeding ulcer. (*B*) Well-attached OTSC tightly grasping a large vessel (*arrow*).

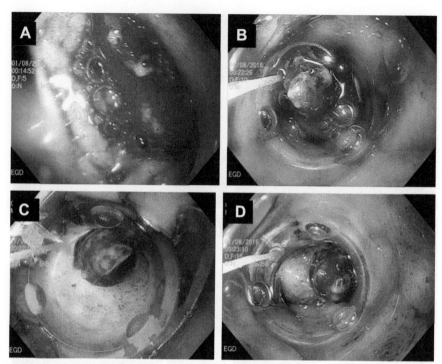

Fig. 3. Key steps to target bleeding lesion with OTSC. (*A*) Approaching the lesion en face. (*B*) Suctioning the lesion. (*C*) Verifying that the target lesion is in the center before releasing the OTSC. (*D*) Successfully released clip.

difficult anatomic locations because of its barrel-shape transparent cap design, which allows suctioning of the bleeding lesion (see **Figs. 2** and **3**). The OTSC system is used in a very similar way to a variceal banding device, which allows for a targeted; that is, en face, approach to the bleeding lesion (see **Fig. 2**). Every endoscopist has encountered bleeding ulcers or lesions that are located in difficult locations and/or positions. Most gastroscopes have the working channel at the 7 o'clock position, making a targeted therapy for lesions located on the posterior or right side of the duodenum or stomach quite difficult; although a previous study demonstrated that using a colonoscope instead of a gastroscope allowed for targeted endoscopic therapy for these lesions because the working channel of the colonoscope is located on the right side.[13] However, having a colonoscope available during emergency NVUGIH is not always

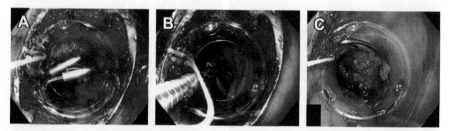

Fig. 4. OTSC in special situations. (*A*) Traditional clip failure. There is ongoing bleeding despite placement of two standard clips. (*B*) The clips are removed. (*C*) An over-the-scope-clip has been placed with successful hemostasis.

Table 2
Endoscopic treatment of nonvariceal gastrointestinal bleeding

Traditional Approach	
Injection	Epinephrine, polidocanol, fibrin glue, Histoacryl
Thermal therapies	Argon plasma coagulation, heater probes, monopolar, bipolar (gold, silver, BICAP [bipolar circum-active probe])
Mechanical	Through the scope clips, endoscopic band ligation
Emerging Treatments	
Injection	Endoscopic ultrasound -guided angiotherapy
Thermal therapies	Coagulation grasper, radiofrequency ablation, cryotherapy
Mechanical	OTSC (Ovesco OTSC, Padlock), suturing system (Apollo) anchor system (prototypes), flexible linear stapler (experimental)
Topical	Hemospray, EndoClot, Pure-Stat, Ankaferd Blood Stopper, oxidized cellulose

feasible. In addition, standard through-the-scope clips often fall off from large, ulcerated, or fibrotic lesions, and may induce more bleeding by lacerating the vessel.

A crucial element to the technical success of OTSC system placement is to accurately position the lesion within the transparent OTSC cap[6,10–16] (see **Fig. 2**). The misapplication of a clip on 1 side of such a lesion may interfere with the successful deployment of a second clip over the defect.[6] Nonetheless, multiple OTSC applications in a single session may still be useful and allow approximation of tissue to facilitate subsequent closure.[6] The authors want to emphasize that careful attention should be paid to suction enough tissue into the cap and to always maintain a clear view of the location of the lumen to avoid inadvertent occlusion of the duodenal lumen. Recently, another clipping device, the Padlock Clip (Aponos Medical, Kingston, NH, USA), which is attached to the scope, became available.[48] The design of this clip is conceptually similar to the OTSC system but the clip is flat and has 6 inner prongs placed in a circumferential fashion.[40] So far, there is only very limited experience with the Padlock system for the treatment of NVUGIH, with only 2 reported cases.[48]

OVER-THE-SCOPE CLIP FOR REFRACTORY PEPTIC ULCER BLEEDING AND OTHER NONVARICEAL UPPER GASTROINTESTINAL HEMORRHAGE

Although the OTSC was first used about 8 years ago to treat NVUGIH, it was not until 2014 that 3 groups published their first studies with this device, focusing on the therapy for refractory NVUGIH.[14–16] The first study was from the University of Alabama at Birmingham, United States; the second from the endoscopy team from Prince of

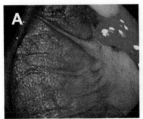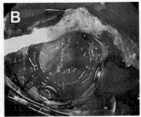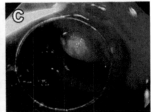

Fig. 5. OTSC for bleeding Dieulafoy lesion (*A–C*).

Wales Hospital, Hong Kong; and the third from the University of Torino, Italy. The first study reported on 12 consecutive subjects (67% men; mean age 59 years, range 29 – 86) with ongoing NVUGIH despite previous traditional endoscopic management. The subjects were quite ill, with a mean American Society of Anesthetists (ASA) score of 3 (range 2– 4), mean hemoglobin of 7.2 g/dL (range 5.2– 9.1), and shock in 75%.[14] They had all received packed red blood cells (mean 5.1 units, range 2 – 12). The cause of bleeding was duodenal ulcer (n = 6), gastric ulcer (n = 2), Dieulafoy lesion (n = 2), anastomotic ulceration (n = 1), and Mallory - Weiss tear (n = 1). Hemostasis with the OTSC was achieved in all subjects. Rebleeding occurred in 2 subjects 1 day and 7 days after OTSC placement, which was stopped with an additional clip. There were no adverse events associated with OTSC.[14] In the study from Hong Kong, Chan and colleagues[15] also used the OTSC for endoscopic control of refractory or major NVUGIH. In that study, 9 subjects (median age 72.5 years, range 39– 91) were included, with bleeding gastric ulcers (n = 2), bleeding duodenal ulcers (n = 5), bleeding gastrointestinal stromal tumor in the stomach (n = 1), and bleeding from ulcerative carcinoma of the pancreas (n = 1). The median size of the ulcers was 2.5 cm. Technical success was achieved in all subjects and the clinical effectiveness was 77.8%. The study from Italy was the largest, including 23 subjects with refractory NVUGIH treated with the OTSC after failure of conventional techniques.[16] The OTSC was effective in 22 out of 23 subjects. One subject required additional emergent selective radiological embolization to stop the hemorrhage.[16] The investigators observed 2 rebleeding episodes at 12 and 24 hours after the procedure; these were successfully treated with additional saline-adrenaline endoscopic injection.[16]

In summary, these 3 studies demonstrated the efficacy and safety of the OTSC to treat subjects with a wide spectrum of causes of NVUGIH in whom traditional methods had failed. Several important aspects should be noted about these studies. First, all subjects had recurrent bleeding despite first-line traditional endoscopic hemostatic approaches. Second, the subjects had large and complex lesions. An advantage of the OTSC is that it can be placed on large and fibrotic lesions, and those with large visible vessels (see **Figs. 3** and **4**). Third, all subjects were treated in tertiary centers by experts in therapeutic endoscopy, which underscores that traditional endoscopic hemostasis may still fail to treat subjects with NVUGIH. Even the OTSC was not 100% effective, with up to 8% rebleeding reported.[14–16] Therefore, OTSC is a useful addition to treat NVUGIH; potentially increasing the effectiveness of endoscopic therapy but there is still a subgroup of subjects (who are likely on anticoagulation) with very complex lesions that mandate additional endoscopic, radiologic, or surgical intervention. These studies seem to show that a single OTSC was able to stop the hemorrhage in most subjects; thus it seems that OTSC may also be considered as first-line therapy (see following discussion).

FIRST-LINE THERAPY FOR PEPTIC ULCER BLEEDING USING THE OVER-THE-SCOPE CLIP

Three important studies on the efficacy of OTSC as first-line therapy in NVUGIH have been published thus far.[11,12,17] Manno and colleagues[17] from Italy treated 40 consecutive subjects (mean age 69 years, range 25–94) with severe NVUGIH with OTSC during a 12-month period. Indications for OTSC treatment included gastric ulcer with a large visible vessel (Forrest IIa; n = 8, 20%), duodenal ulcer (Forrest Ib; n = 7, 18%), duodenal ulcer with large visible vessel (Forrest IIa; n = 6, 15%), Dieulafoy lesion (n = 6, 15%) and other secondary indications (n = 13, 32%). Technical success and primary hemostasis were achieved in all subjects (100%). No rebleeding, need for surgical or radiological embolization treatment, or other adverse events were observed during the 30-day follow-up period.[17] In a study from Germany, Richter-Schrag and colleagues[11] identified all subjects with UGIH and lower gastrointestinal bleeding in a tertiary care endoscopic referral center who underwent OTSC as first-line or second-line therapy. Primary hemostasis and clinical success was achieved in 88 out of 100 (88%) and 78 out of 100 (78%) subjects, respectively. The failure rate was significantly lower when OTSC was applied as first-line endoscopic therapy compared with second-line endoscopic therapy (4.9% vs 23%, P = .008).[11] From Germany, in the largest study published to date, Wedi and colleagues[12] studied 118 subjects with NVUGIH undergoing endoscopic hemostasis with OTSC as first-line endoscopic therapy. In total, 118 subjects with a median age of 73.5 years (range 29–93 years) were included. The distribution of subjects with respect to risk category revealed a median Rockall score of 7 (range 3–10). Successful primary hemostasis was achieved in 92.4%. An advantage if this study was the utilization of the Rockall score and comparison with various risk groups based on Rockall score. The investigators found that rebleeding or continued bleeding was more common in subjects with high-risk Rockall score (21.4%) compared with low-risk subjects (4.9%).[12] When comparing OTSC as first-line therapy with subjects in moderate-risk and high-risk groups, the differences in rebleeding were quite striking. The occurrence of rebleeding or continued bleeding was significantly lower in the moderate-risk group (Rockall risk score 4–7) with 4.9%, as well as in the high-risk group (Rockall risk score $\geq$8) with 21.4%, compared with the Rockall cohort 24.0% and 53.2%, respectively (P<.001). In summary, this study showed that first-line endoscopic therapy with OTSC is effective and safe, seems superior to standard care, and that first-line endoscopic therapy with OTSC significantly reduces rebleeding and rebleeding-associated mortality in NVUGIH.

These data show that OTSC has become a useful and valid initial or first-line therapy for NVUGIH. Whereas the arguments are quite strong to use OTSC as a first-line therapy in high-risk patients or lesions, its ease of use and effectiveness are paving its way to become a first-line therapy in most NVUGIH episodes. In the authors' experience it does not make sense to be placing multiple through-the-scope clips on a large or fibrotic lesion, or on an ulcer with a large visible vessel (see **Fig. 1**). First, this approach is cumbersome, time-consuming, more expensive, and likely more risky because a traditional though-the-scope clip may lacerate the vessel or lesion, in contrast to the OTSC, which entraps the vessel or bleeding lesion (see **Figs. 2–5**). Approaching these lesions with a simple and easy method such as OTSC may result in better technical success, improved patient outcomes, and less expense.[11–22] Indeed, a recent study evaluating 262 clip applications showed that implementation of OTSC is easy, feasible, and effective during routine endoscopic practice.[22]

HEMOSPRAY

Hemospray TC325 (Cook Medical Inc, Winston-Salem, NC, USA) is a novel, hemostatic powder that has been developed for gastrointestinal use.[23–31] The powder is thought to achieve hemostasis by concentrating clotting factors and forming a mechanical plug on the injured blood vessel.[23,24] Holster and colleagues[23] studied the hemostatic mode of action of Hemospray on coagulation and clot formation both in vitro and in vivo by using recalcification time, thromboelastometry, and plasma coagulation tests (activated partial thromboplastin time and prothrombin time) on blood samples mixed with Hemospray, and compared this with talcum powder (negative control) and kaolin (positive control). Then the investigators performed scanning electron microscopy and light microscopy on in vitro thrombi and on gastric thrombi from an animal model of gastrointestinal hemorrhage treated with Hemospray. They found that the median recalcification time of whole blood was 187.5 seconds. The addition of 1 mg/mL and 10 mg/mL of Hemospray significantly shortened this time (median 60 and 45 seconds, respectively, $P < .05$). The median clotting time of whole blood was 160 seconds and this was also significantly reduced by the addition of Hemospray to 91 seconds ($P = .005$). The plasma prothrombin time of 11.6 seconds was significantly reduced by Hemospray (9.5 seconds, $P = .011$). Electron microscopy of in vivo clots demonstrated that Hemospray rapidly interacted with whole blood, forming a confluent mass over the bleeding site. This study shows that Hemospray has an initial mechanical effect, covering the bleeding site, followed by enhanced clot formation in vivo and shortened coagulation time in vitro.

HEMOSPRAY IN NONVARICEAL UPPER GASTROINTESTINAL HEMORRHAGE

Although the topical hemostatic powder Hemospray is currently categorized as emerging endoscopic therapy, there are several studies documenting its efficacy and, in some countries, similar to what we have seen with OTSC, it is considered standard endoscopic therapy.

Hemospray was first widely used in Asia. Indeed, we were given the opportunity to apply Hemospray for bleeding gastroduodenal ulcers during the Hong Kong Live Endoscopy course in 2011 (Klaus Mönkemüller, http://www.hksde.org/wp2011/v06-E_Haemospray.wmv). In parallel, its use was becoming widespread in Europe in countries such as the United Kingdom, Croatia, and The Netherlands. In a prospective pilot study by Sung and colleagues,[24] 20 consecutive adults (18 men, 2 women; mean age 60.2 years) with confirmed peptic ulcer bleeding (Forrest score Ia or Ib) underwent upper gastrointestinal endoscopy and application of Hemospray within 24 hours of hospital admission once hemodynamically stable. Acute hemostasis was achieved in 95% (19/20) of subjects; 1 subject had a pseudoaneurysm requiring arterial embolization. Bleeding recurred in 2 subjects within 72 hours (demonstrated by hemoglobin drop); neither had active bleeding identified at the 72-hour endoscopy. No mortality, major adverse events, or treatment-related or procedure-related serious adverse events were reported.[24] Holster and colleagues[25] further evaluated the utility of Hemospray in anticoagulated subjects. A total of 16 unselected consecutive subjects with UGIH who were treated with Hemospray were analyzed (8 taking antithrombotic therapy [ATT] for various indications and 8 not using ATT). Initial hemostasis was achieved after Hemospray application in 5 out of 8 subjects on ATT (63%) and in all 8 subjects not on ATT ($P = .20$). Rebleeding rates were similar between groups. These preliminary data on the use of Hemospray in the management of UGIH were promising in both subjects with and without ATT use.[25]

Sinha and colleagues[26] also reported on the use of Hemospray as an adjunctive agent in subjects with high-risk Forrest Ia and Ib lesions. A total of 20 subjects (median age 75 years, 50% men, 60% Forrest Ia ulcer) were treated with Hemospray as a second agent to adrenaline, or as an adjunct to the combination of adrenaline with either clips or a thermal device. Primary hemostasis was attained in 95%, with an overall rebleeding rate at 7 days of 16%. This study showed that Hemospray seemed promising as an adjunct to conventional hemostasis methods for NVUGIH.[26]

In a retrospective study, Yau and colleagues[27] treated 19 subjects with various causes of NVUGIH with Hemospray. The lesions included peptic ulcers in 12 (63.2%) subjects, Dieulafoy lesions in 2 (10.5%), mucosal erosion in 1 (5.3%), angiodysplastic lesions in 1 (5.3%), ampullectomy in 1 (5.3%), polypectomy in 1 (5.3%), and an unidentified lesion in 1 (5.3%). Hemospray was administered as monotherapy in 2 (10.5%) subjects, first-line modality in 1 (5.3%), and as a rescue modality in

16 (84.2%). Hemospray was applied prophylactically to nonbleeding lesions in 4 (21.1%) subjects and therapeutically to bleeding lesions in 15 (78.9%). Acute hemostasis was achieved in 14 out of 15 (93.3%) subjects. Rebleeding within 7 days occurred in 7 out of 18 (38.9%) subjects.[27] This study showed that Hemospray might be used in high-risk cases as a temporizing measure or as a bridge toward more definitive therapy.[27]

In a large multicenter study, Smith and colleagues[28] evaluated 63 subjects (44 men, 19 women), median age 69 (range 21–98) years, with NVUGIH requiring endoscopic hemostasis who were treated with Hemospray TC-325. There were 30 subjects with bleeding ulcers and 33 with other NVUGIH lesions. Fifty-five (87%) subjects were treated with TC-325 as monotherapy, with 47 out of 55 (85.5%) achieving primary hemostasis, and the rebleeding rate at 7 days was 15%. The primary hemostasis rate for TC-325 for inhospital subjects with ulcer bleeds was 76%. Eight subjects, who otherwise may have required either surgery or interventional radiology, were treated with TC-325 as second-line therapy after failure of other endoscopic treatments, all of whom achieved hemostasis following the adjunct use of TC-325.[28]

In a smaller study involving 16 subjects, Sulz and colleagues[29] also reported that Hemospray was useful and effective as a treatment option in GIB in everyday clinical practice. From Canada, Chen and colleagues[30] reported on a larger cohort, including 60 subjects receiving 67 treatments with Hemospray. Their study included 21 with nonmalignant NVUGIH and 19 with malignant upper gastrointestinal bleeding.[29] Immediate hemostasis was achieved in 66 cases (98.5%), with 6 cases (9.5%) of early rebleeding. A novel finding of this study is the demonstration of Hemospray effectiveness for subjects with malignant upper GI hemorrhage.[30]

Finally, the largest study on Hemospray so far is from France.[31] A total of 202 subjects were enrolled and 64 endoscopists participated from 20 centers.[31] Hemospray TC-325 was used as salvage therapy in 108 subjects (53.5%). The cause of bleeding was ulcer in 75 subjects (37.1%), tumor in 61 (30.2%), postendoscopic therapy in 35 (17.3%), or other in 31 (15.3%). Application of the hemostatic powder was found to be very easy or easy in 31.7% and 55.4%, respectively. The immediate efficacy rate was 96.5%. Recurrence of UGIH was noted at day 8 and day 30 in 26.7% and 33.5%, respectively.[31] This large study is important because it shows that Hemospray is easy to use, is safe, and seems to be effective.[31] In addition, it seems that Hemospray is a cost-effective therapy as shown in a decision analysis.[32]

OTHER EMERGING THERAPIES

There is an increasing spectrum of emerging therapies for NVUGIH (see **Table 2**).[33–41] However, there is generally a lack of larger case series or studies. Therefore, this article only briefly discusses these therapies because they remain either theoretic or performed only at specific institutions, and may never truly emerge to play a role in the endoscopic therapy for NVUGIH.

ENDOSCOPIC ULTRASOUND-GUIDED ANGIOGRAPHY

In an interesting study several years ago, Fockens and colleagues[33] used endosonography to detect endoscopically nonvisible Dieulafoy lesions of the upper GI tract. In 3 subjects, sclerotherapy was accomplished under endoscopic ultrasound (EUS)-guidance.[33] Since then only a handful of case reports have been reported on the potential use of EUS-guided angiographic intervention. Nevertheless, the results are not easily reproducible and the use of EUS as an interventional tool for managing NVUGIH has remained limited to a few centers worldwide.[33,34]

RADIOFREQUENCY ABLATION

RFA is an accepted therapy to treat Barrett's esophagus with dysplasia.[35] However, owing to its thermal destruction capabilities, it has been also been used to treat various bleeding lesions, most commonly gastric antral vascular ectasias (GAVE).[36] The traditional endoscopic treatment of GAVE is argon plasma coagulation but results are not always positive. RFA is a new endoscopic therapy that may be an attractive option for the treatment of GAVE. In an open-label, retrospective, case series, Dray and colleagues[36] treated a total of 24 subjects with GAVE using RFA. The mean number of PRBC transfusions significantly decreased in all 23 transfusion-dependent subjects, from a mean of 10.6, plus or minus 12.1, during the 6 months before RFA, to a mean of 2.5, plus or minus 5.9, during the 6 months following RFA treatment ($P<.001$); 15 subjects (65.2%) were weaned off blood transfusions completely. All subjects had a significant increase in hemoglobin after RFA therapy. This study showed that RFA for the treatment of GAVE seems feasible and safe, and it significantly reduced the need for RBC transfusion and increased hemoglobin levels.[36] Additional studies or case reports using RFA for acute NVUGIH are lacking.

EndoClot

EndoClot is a novel topical hemostatic powder approved for use in NVUGIH. The EndoClot application system consists of 2 g of powder within a mixing chamber, which is applied through a 2300-mm delivery catheter fed through the working channel of an endoscope.[37] An external air compressor creates the sustained force required to drive the powder from within the chamber through the catheter, resulting in the multidirectional distribution of the product onto the mucosa.[37] Given the wide field of distribution, an en face view of the point of bleeding is not essential. This is particularly useful for lesions that are difficult to access, such as ulcers located on the posterior duodenal wall. In a retrospective study, Beg and colleagues[37] treated 21 subjects with EndoClot and found a hemostatic efficacy of 100%. EndoClot was used as a second agent in 7 cases, a third agent in 9 cases, and the fourth form of endoscopic therapy in 5 cases. The lesions treated included duodenal ulcer (n = 14), Mallory-Weiss tear (n = 2), gastric ulcer (n = 2), malignancy (n = 1), esophageal ulcer (n = 1), and nonspecific gastric oozing (n = 1).[37] Prei and colleagues[38] performed a prospective open-label study of EndoClot for various types of NVUGIH. Seventy subjects with acute GI bleeding were recruited into the study, of which 83% had upper GI hemorrhage.[38] Treatment success was achieved in 64% of cases in which it was used as rescue therapy.[38] Rebleeding occurred in 11% (8/70), in 10% EndoClot served as a bridge to surgery (7/70).[38] This study showed that EndoClot is an additional tool in the setting of NVUGIH and it can be used as monotherapy or in combination with other hemostasis modalities. Furthermore, in a few cases, the use of EndoClot served as a bridge to surgery when standard methods of endoscopic hemostasis failed. Whether this topical hemostatic powder will have significant clinical applicability remains to be proven because its costs are high. Nevertheless, its ease of application and usefulness for diffuse bleeding lesions make this agent and Hemospray attractive adjunctive treatments on the emergency bleeding cart.

ENDOSCOPIC BAND LIGATION

Endoscopic band ligation (EBL) is an established method to treat various types of NVUGIH lesions. However, recently, EBL has been proven quite efficacious for the therapy for GAVE.[39] In the only prospective study thus far, Zepeda-Gómez and colleagues[39] enrolled 21 consecutive subjects with GAVE and applied multiple EBLs in the stomach. A clinical response was achieved in 19 subjects (91%). A significant improvement in the mean hemoglobin level was noted after EBL ($P < .001$) and a significant decrease in blood transfusion requirements per month ($P = .001$). No major adverse events were observed during the study period. The mean follow-up was 10 months. The investigators found that EBL is an effective and safe treatment of GAVE.

CRYOTHERAPY

Cryotherapy has been proposed as a useful method to provide hemostasis in diffusely bleeding NVUGIH. However, cryotherapy has never reached the clinical stage of routine use. Nevertheless, it is worth mentioning that data are emerging to show its potential use in specific conditions such as GAVE.[40] Cho and colleagues, from Canada, assessed the efficacy and safety of cryotherapy for the endoscopic treatment of GAVE. Subjects received 3 sessions of endoscopic cryotherapy at 3 to 6 week intervals and had a follow-up endoscopy 4 weeks thereafter. Overall, 12 subjects ranging in age from 43 to 89 years were enrolled. Six subjects (50%) had a complete response and 6 subjects had a partial response. The mean number of units of blood transfused in the period of 3 months before cryotherapy and during the 3-month follow-up period was 4.6 and 1.7 units, respectively. An increased mean hemoglobin level, from 9.9 to 11.3 g/dL, was noted. The mean duration of the cryotherapy was 5 minutes (range 1–15 minutes). This pilot study showed that endoscopic cryotherapy seemed to be a safe and effective treatment of GAVE.[40] The authors are unsure whether its use will disseminate beyond specific tertiary centers because the setup for cryotherapy is not available in most endoscopic centers worldwide.

SURGICAL HEMOSTATIC AGENTS (ANKAFERD, OXIDIZED CELLULOSE)

Ankaferd Blood Stopper (ABS) is a topical hemostatic agent of herbal origin that has been used for a long time in Anatolia, Turkey, but has only recently become available for routine clinical use in dermatologic and dental surgery.[41] Ankaferd is a standardized mixture of the plants *Thymus vulgaris* (thyme-dried herbal extract), *Glycyrrhiza glabra* (licorice-dried leaf extract), *Vitis vinifera* (grape-dried leaf extract), *Alpinia officinarum* (lesser galangal-dried leaf extract), and *Urtica dioica* (stinging nettle-dried root extract). It forms a clot by precipitating fibrinogen and forming a protein network that acts as an anchor for erythrocyte aggregation.[41,42] The topical use of ABS has been approved by the Turkish Ministry of Health for the management of dermal, external postsurgical, and postdental surgery bleeding.[41,42] In a prospective study, 27 subjects with various causes of NVUGIH were treated with ABS.[42] The hemostasis rate was 73%. ABS seemed particularly useful for diffusely bleeding lesions. In addition, ABS could be used as a secondary, combination or rescue therapy in difficult cases of NVUGIH.

Oxidized regenerated cellulose (ORC) is a widely available surgical hemostatic material. ORC can be considered a topical hemostatic agent. The mechanism of action of ORC is still unclear but data show that it activates platelets and provides mechanical hemostasis by dehydrating or sponge-like mechanisms.[43] Indeed, ORC is generally used for heavy bleeding because it has a high absorptive capacity resulting from its dense fibrous composition; ORC can absorb up to 7 times its physiologic weight.[43] An in vivo, prospective, proof-of-concept study, demonstrated that ORC is effective in achieving hemostasis after endoscopic resection in heparinized rabbits.[43] Since then, 2 case reports have shown that cellulose is a useful adjunct in massive NVUGIH, once to treat a recalcitrant anastomotic ulcer and the other to treat hemosuccus pancreaticus.[44,45]

ENDOSCOPIC SUTURING DEVICES

Data are lacking on the use of suturing devices such as the OverStitch (Apollo Endosurgery, Inc, Austin, TX) for managing acute NVUGIH.[46,47] Although the concept of oversewing a lesion through an endoscope is appealing, device limitations, such as the technical complexity and the need for a specialized double-channel endoscope, impaired visibility in the setting of active bleeding, and restricted maneuverability and access to certain anatomic locations of the upper GI tract, have limited the use of this suturing system in the acute setting. However, the device seems well-suited to manage chronic blood loss resulting from anastomotic ulcers and for the prevention of delayed bleeding following endoscopic mucosal resection or endoscopic submucosal dissection.[46,47]

REFERENCES

1. Jovanovic I, Vormbrock K, Wilcox CM, et al. Therapeutic and interventional endoscopy for gastrointestinal bleeding. Eur J Trauma Emerg Surg 2011;11:301–22.
2. Mönkemüller KE, Eloubeidi M. Bleeding peptic ulcer: what's new? Gastrointest Endosc 2002;56:157–9.
3. Gölder SK, Brückner J, Messmann H. Endoscopic hemostasis state of the art - Nonvariceal bleeding. World J Gastrointest Endosc 2016;8(4):205–11.
4. Gralnek IM, Barkun AN, Bardou M. Management of acute bleeding from a peptic ulcer. N Engl J Med 2008;359:928–37.
5. Aabakken L. Current endoscopic and pharmacological therapy of peptic ulcer bleeding. Best Pract Res Clin Gastroenterol 2008;22:243–59.
6. Mönkemüller K, Peter S, Toshniwal J, et al. Multipurpose use of the 'bear claw' (over-the-scope-clip system) to treat endoluminal gastrointestinal disorders. Dig Endosc 2014;26(3):350–7.
7. Mönkemüller K, Toshniwal J, Zabielski M. Utility of the "bear claw", or over-the-scope clip (OTSC) system, to provide endoscopic hemostasis for bleeding posterior duodenal ulcers. Endoscopy 2012;44(Suppl 2 UCTN):E412–3.
8. Vormbrock K, Zabielski M, Mönkemüller K. Use of the "bear claw" (over-the-scope-clip) to achieve hemostasis of a large gastric ulcer with bleeding visible vessel. Gastrointest Endosc 2012;76(4):917–8.
9. Sulz MC, Bertolini R, Frei R, et al. Multipurpose use of the over-the-scope-clip system ("Bear claw") in the gastrointestinal tract: Swiss experience in a tertiary center. World J Gastroenterol 2014;20(43):16287–92.
10. Mudumbi S, Velazquez-Aviña J, Neumann H, et al. Anchoring of self-expanding metal stents using the over-the-scope clip, and a technique for subsequent removal. Endoscopy 2014;46:1106–9.
11. Richter-Schrag HJ, Glatz T, Walker C, et al. First-line endoscopic treatment with over-the-scope clips significantly improves the primary failure and rebleeding rates in high-risk gastrointestinal bleeding: A single-center experience with 100 cases. World J Gastroenterol 2016;22(41):9162–71.
12. Wedi E, Fischer A, Hochberger J, et al. Multicenter evaluation of first-line endoscopic treatment with the OTSC in acute non-variceal upper gastrointestinal bleeding and comparison with the Rockall cohort: the FLETRock study. Surg Endosc 2017. https://doi.org/10.1007/s00464-017-5678-7.

13. Mönkemüller K, Neumann H, Bellutti M, et al. Use of a colonoscope to perform endoscopic therapy in patients with active bleeding from posterior duodenal and gastric ulcers. Endoscopy 2009;41(Suppl 2):E93–4.

14. Skinner M, Gutierrez JP, Neumann H, et al. Over-the-scope clip placement is effective rescue therapy for severe acute upper gastrointestinal bleeding. Endosc Int Open 2014;2:E37–40.

15. Chan SM, Chiu PW, Teoh AY, et al. Use of the over-the-scope clip for treatment of refractory upper gastrointestinal bleeding: a case series. Endoscopy 2014;46(5): 428–31.

16. Manta R, Galloro G, Mangiavillano B, et al. Over-the-scope clip (OTSC) represents an effective endoscopic treatment for acute GI bleeding after failure of conventional techniques. Surg Endosc 2013;27(9):3162–4.

17. Manno M, Mangiafico S, Caruso A, et al. First-line endoscopic treatment with OTSC in patients with high-risk non-variceal upper gastrointestinal bleeding: preliminary experience in 40 cases. Surg Endosc 2016;30(5):2026–9.

18. Wedi E, von Renteln D, Gonzalez S, et al. Use of the over-the-scope-clip (OTSC) in non-variceal upper gastrointestinal bleeding in patients with severe cardiovascular comorbidities: a retrospective study. Endosc Int Open 2017;5(9):E875–82.

19. Douaihy Y, Kesavan M, Deeb L, et al. Over-the-scope clip to the rescue of a bleeding gastroduodenal artery pseudoaneurysm. Gastrointest Endosc 2016; 84(5):854–5.

20. Fujihara S, Mori H, Kobara H, et al. Use of an over-the-scope clip and a colonoscope for complete hemostasis of a duodenal diverticular bleed. Endoscopy 2015;47(Suppl 1 UCTN):E236–7.

21. Lamberts R, Koch A, Binner C, et al. Use of over-the-scope clips (OTSC) for hemostasis in gastrointestinal bleeding in patients under antithrombotic therapy. Endosc Int Open 2017;5(5):E324–30.

22. Honegger C, Valli PV, Wiegand N, et al. Establishment of over-the-scope-clips (OTSC®) in daily endoscopic routine. United European Gastroenterol J 2017; 5(2):247–54.

23. Holster IL, van Beusekom HM, Kuipers EJ, et al. Effects of a hemostatic powder hemospray on coagulation and clot formation. Endoscopy 2015;47(7):638–45.

24. Sung JJ, Luo D, Wu JC, et al. Early clinical experience of the safety and effectiveness of Hemospray in achieving hemostasis in patients with acute peptic ulcer bleeding. Endoscopy 2011;43(4):291–5.

25. Holster IL, Kuipers EJ, Tjwa ET. Hemospray in the treatment of upper gastrointestinal hemorrhage in patients on antithrombotic therapy. Endoscopy 2013;45(1): 63–6.

26. Sinha R, Lockman KA, Church NI, et al. The use of hemostatic spray as an adjunct to conventional hemostatic measures in high-risk nonvariceal upper GI bleeding (with video). Gastrointest Endosc 2016;84(6):900–6.

27. Yau AH, Ou G, Galorport C, et al. Safety and efficacy of Hemospray® in upper gastrointestinal bleeding. Can J Gastroenterol Hepatol 2014;28(2):72–6.

28. Smith LA, Stanley AJ, Bergman JJ, et al. Hemospray application in nonvariceal upper gastrointestinal bleeding: results of the survey to evaluate the application of hemospray in the luminal tract. J Clin Gastroenterol 2014;48(10):e89–92.

29. Sulz MC, Frei R, Meyenberger C, et al. Routine use of hemospray for gastrointestinal bleeding: prospective two-center experience in Switzerland. Endoscopy 2014;46(7):619–24.

30. Chen YI, Barkun A, Nolan S. Hemostatic powder TC-325 in the management of upper and lower gastrointestinal bleeding: a two-year experience at a single institution. Endoscopy 2015;47(2):167–71.
31. Haddara S, Jacques J, Lecleire S, et al. A novel hemostatic powder for upper gastrointestinal bleeding: a multicenter study (the "GRAPHE" registry). Endoscopy 2016;48(12):1084–95.
32. Barkun AN, Adam V, Lu Y, et al. Using hemospray improves the cost-effectiveness ratio in the management of upper gastrointestinal nonvariceal bleeding. J Clin Gastroenterol 2018;52(1):36–44.
33. Fockens P, Meenan J, van Dullemen HM, et al. Dieulafoy's disease: endosonographic detection and endosonography-guided treatment. Gastrointest Endosc 1996;44:437–42.
34. Mathew S, Zacharias P, Kumar L, et al. Duodenal arteriovenous malformation: endosonographic diagnosis and coil embolization. Endoscopy 2016;48(S 01):E378–9.
35. Mönkemüller K. Radiofrequency ablation for Barrett esophagus with confirmed low-grade dysplasia. JAMA 2014;311(12):1205–6.
36. Dray X, Repici A, Gonzalez P, et al. Radiofrequency ablation for the treatment of gastric antral vascular ectasia. Endoscopy 2014;46:963–9.
37. Beg S, Al-Bakir I, Bhuva M, et al. Early clinical experience of the safety and efficacy of EndoClot in the management of non-variceal upper gastrointestinal bleeding. Endosc Int Open 2015;3(6):E605–9.
38. Prei JC, Barmeyer C, Bürgel N, et al. EndoClot polysaccharide hemostatic system in nonvariceal gastrointestinal bleeding: results of a prospective multicente observational pilot study. J Clin Gastroenterol 2016;50(10):e95–100.
39. Zepeda-Gómez S, Sultanian R, Teshima C, et al. Gastric antral vascular ectasia: a prospective study of treatment with endoscopic band ligation. Endoscopy 2015;47(6):538–40.
40. Cho S, Zanati S, Yong E, et al. Endoscopic cryotherapy for the management of gastric antral vascular ectasia. Gastrointest Endosc 2008;68:895–902.
41. Kurt M, Kacar S, Onal IK, et al. Ankaferd Blood Stopper as an effective adjunctive hemostatic agent for the management of life-threatening arterial bleeding of the digestive tract. Endoscopy 2008;40(Suppl 2):E262.
42. Beyazit Y, Kekilli M, Haznedaroglu IC, et al. Ankaferd hemostat in the management of gastrointestinal hemorrhages. World J Gastroenterol 2011;17:3962–70.
43. Velázquez-Aviña J, Mönkemüller K, Sakai P, et al. Hemostatic effect of oxidized regenerated cellulose in an experimental gastric mucosal resection model. Endoscopy 2014;46(10):878–82.
44. Skinner M, Velazquez-Avina J, Mönkemüller K. Overtube-assisted endoscopic application of oxidized cellulose to achieve hemostasis in anastomotic ulcer bleeding. Gastrointest Endosc 2014;80(5):917–8.
45. Ruiz-Tovar J, Oller I, Barreras JA, et al. Exceptional use of a surgical oxidized cellulose polymer taponade in a patient with hemosuccus pancreaticus. Cir Esp 2015;93(1):47–8.
46. Jirapinyo P, Watson RR, Thompson C. Use of a novel endoscopic suturing device to treat recalcitrant marginal ulceration (with video). Gastrointest Endosc 2012;76:435–9.
47. ASGE Technology Committee, Bhat YM, Banerjee S, Barth BA, et al. Endoscopic closure devices. Gastrointest Endosc 2012;76:244–51.
48. Dinelli M, Omazzi B, Andreozzi P, et al. First clinical experiences with a novel endoscopic over-the-scope clip system. Endosc Int Open 2017;5(3):E151–6.

The Cutting Edge
Doppler Probe in Guiding Endoscopic Hemostasis

Kevin A. Ghassemi, MD[a,b,]*, Dennis M. Jensen, MD[a,b,c]

KEYWORDS

- Upper gastrointestinal bleeding • Colonic diverticular hemorrhage
- Endoscopic risk stratification • Doppler endoscopic probe
- Gastrointestinal hemostasis

KEY POINTS

- GI bleeding is a significant health burden, with peptic ulcers and diverticular hemorrhage being the most common upper and lower GI causes.
- Assessment of impact on interventions for GI bleeding are based on several clinical outcomes, including primary hemostasis and rebleeding rates, length of hospitalization, and need for red blood cell transfusion.
- The doppler endoscopic probe (DEP) can be used for risk stratification and a guide to definitive hemostasis in non-variceal upper GI and colonic diverticular hemorrhage.

INTRODUCTION

Gastrointestinal (GI) bleeding continues to be a significant health and economic burden. Over the past 2 decades there has been a decline in hospitalization for nonvariceal upper GI (NVUGI) hemorrhage as well as a reduction in NVUGI bleeding–associated mortality. Concurrently, there has been an increase in the use of inpatient upper endoscopy—including early endoscopy—and endoscopic therapy.[1] Peptic ulcers are still the most common cause of NVUGI hemorrhage.[2] Although most patients with acute lower GI (LGI) bleeding stop bleeding spontaneously, morbidity and mortality are higher in older patients and those with comorbid medical conditions.[3] Diverticular hemorrhage is the most common etiology of severe LGI bleeding that requires hospitalization.[4]

Disclosure Statement: The CURE research included was partially supported by a clinical Veterans Administration Merit Review grant 5I01CX001403-02 (D.M. Jensen, PI) and NIH-NIDDK CURE-DDRC grant DK41301 (Human Studies Core). D.M. Jensen is on the speakers' bureau for Boston Scientific Corporation and is a consultant for Vascular Technology Inc.
[a] Vatche and Tamar Manoukian Division of Digestive Diseases, David Geffen School of Medicine at UCLA, 100 Medical Plaza Driveway, Los Angeles, CA 90095, USA; [b] CURE: Digestive Diseases Research Center, 11301 Wilshire Boulevard, Los Angeles, CA 90073, USA; [c] Department of Medicine, VA West Los Angeles Medical Center, 11301 Wilshire Boulevard, Los Angeles, CA 90073, USA
* Corresponding author. 100 UCLA Medical Plaza #205, Los Angeles, CA 90095.
E-mail address: kghassemi@mednet.ucla.edu

Gastrointest Endoscopy Clin N Am 28 (2018) 321–330
https://doi.org/10.1016/j.giec.2018.02.005
1052-5157/18/© 2018 Elsevier Inc. All rights reserved.

Several endoscopic techniques are available to treat bleeding from focal GI lesions. It has been difficult to demonstrate, however, a mortality improvement. Therefore, other clinical outcomes—primary hemostasis rates, rebleeding rates, length of hospitalization, need for red blood cell transfusions, and rate of other interventions, such as angiographic embolization or surgery—are used to assess the effects of interventions. This article examines Doppler endoscopic probe (DEP) for risk stratification and as a guide to definitive hemostasis of NVUGI bleeding (eg, ulcers, Dieulafoy lesions and Mallory-Weiss tears) and colonic diverticular hemorrhage. This article also reports the importance of residual arterial blood flow underneath stigmata of recent hemorrhage (SRH) as a significant risk factor for rebleeding and worse outcomes after standard, visually guided endoscopic hemostasis of nonvariceal GI lesions.

ENDOSCOPIC APPROACH TO UPPER GASTROINTESTINAL BLEEDING
Pre-endoscopic Setting

Patients with severe or ongoing upper GI (UGI) hemorrhage (ie, high-volume, bloody gastric lavage or ongoing hematemesis, melena, or hematochezia) should undergo urgent endoscopy soon after hemodynamic resuscitation, usually in an ICU or monitored bed unit. Based on a large national study, those with significant comorbidities (American Anesthesiology Association [ASA] scores $\geq$3) are reported to have the lowest mortality when urgent esophagogastroduodenoscopies (EGDs) are performed in a range of 10 hours to 18 hours after admission and resuscitation.[5] This is the safest window in high-risk patients for performing urgent EGD, provided patients are adequately resuscitated. In contrast, hemodynamically stable patients with low ASA scores of 1 to 2 and with severe UGI bleeding can undergo endoscopy within 24 hours without increasing their mortality.[5] For severe UGI bleeding, therapeutic channel endoscopes with a large-diameter suction channel are useful for removal of fresh blood and clots from the UGI tract during urgent endoscopy. Additionally, a water pump for targeted irrigation of lesions is useful to facilitate suctioning of diluted blood and good visualization of ulcers and other focal lesions.

Endoscopic Evaluation and Risk Stratification

In addition to diagnosing UGI lesions, an endoscopist should categorize SRH because these predict the risk of lesion rebleeding. The Forrest classification has been used in Asia, the United Kingdom, and Europe to classify ulcers with stigmata according to risk of rebleeding.[6,7] In contrast, descriptive classifications are used in the United States. Considered together, these are active spurting bleeding (Forrest IA), oozing bleeding (Forrest IB), pigmented protuberance or nonbleeding visible vessel (NBVV) (Forrest IIA), adherent clot (Forrest IIb), flat pigmented spot (Forrest IIC), and clean-based ulcer (Forrest III). Patients at the highest risk of rebleeding without endoscopic treatment are those with spurting arterial bleeding—Forrest IA treated medically (90% rebleed rate), NBVV—Forrest IIA (50% rebleed), or adherent clot—Forrest IIB (33% rebleed).[8,9] These patients and those with the intermediate-risk stigmata of oozing bleeding and flat spots with arterial flow underneath,[7,9–11] benefit from endoscopic hemostasis, whereas low-risk patients with a flat spot without arterial flow detected underneath or clean ulcer base do not according to current clinical guidelines and recent randomized controlled trial (RCT) DEP studies.[8,9,12]

Doppler Endoscopic Probe

The DEP for detecting arterial blood flow underneath SRH during GI endoscopy was first described in 1982.[13] Currently, the DEP monitoring equipment has been simplified and is easy to teach GI endoscopists how to use.[7,14] The DEP catheter is approximately 2 mm in diameter and can be passed through the suction channel of any diagnostic or therapeutic upper endoscope or colonoscope (**Fig. 1**). The technique was most commonly described for bleeding ulcers, but any focal GI lesion can be interrogated. The base of an ulcer should first be flushed with target irrigation to remove any blood, clots, debris, or exudate. After lubricating the tip (with water-soluble lubricant), the DEP catheter is passed and applied to the ulcer base with light pressure at multiple points, adjacent to the SRH and moving outward (**Fig. 2**). The underlying artery in ulcers moves away from the visual SRH in a straight line.[7,9] By mapping in 4 quadrants straight out from the SRH, the direction of the artery (relative to the stigmata) and the depth can be determined with the DEP. For ulcers, the superficial setting ($\leq$1.5 mm) usually detects underlying blood flow and less commonly the middle setting on the control unit is used ($\leq$4 mm). The endoscopist should realize that the underlying artery is the closest to the ulcer base at the SRH and that the artery may dive abruptly while moving away from the SRH.[7,9] According to Doppler principles, a tangential application is needed to detect blood flow rather than a perpendicular approach.[13–15] For nonvariceal lesions, the blood flow detected is arterial and not venous. On the current unit used in the United States, a positive DEP signal is detected as an audible swish-swish sound indicative of pulsatile blood flow.[7,14]

DEP is particularly valuable in predicting the initial risk of rebleeding in peptic ulcer bleeding (PUB), where to target endoscopic hemostasis, and then to assess success of endoscopic treatment. Because residual underlying arterial blood flow determines lesion rebleeding after visually guided hemostasis, DEP can serve as a guide for application of additional endoscopic treatment to achieve definitive hemostasis. See **Fig. 3** for an example of hemoclip placement next to the SRH to target the underlying artery for mechanical closure of it.

Prospective studies of patients with PUB have reported the importance of arterial blood flow as a risk factor for rebleeding. In a study of 52 patients undergoing DEP, 23 underwent endoscopic therapy. Twelve patients had a positive DEP signal prior to endoscopic therapy. Of those, 9 (75%) were converted to a negative DEP signal after endoscopic therapy. Three patients with a persistent DEP-positive signal rebled within 30 days compared with only 1 patient (11%) whose ulcer was converted to a DEP-negative signal.[14,15] In a more recent study, 163 patients with severe PUB underwent DEP evaluation during urgent endoscopy.[7] Patients with major SRH (spurting arterial bleeding—Forrest IA, NBVV—Forrest IIA, and adherent clot—Forrest IIB) had a significantly higher DEP positive rate for arterial blood flow (on EGD before hemostasis) than intermediate SRH (oozing alone—Forrest IB or flat spot—Forrest III):

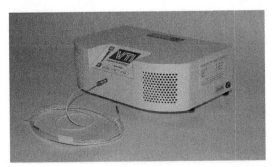

Fig. 1. DEP control unit and catheter. (*Courtesy of* Vascular Technology Inc, Nashua, NH; with permission.)

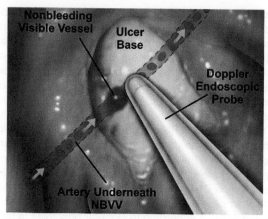

Fig. 2. DEP interrogation of an ulcer base with an NBVV.

87% versus 42%, respectively. After standard visually guided endoscopic hemostasis with either thermal probe or hemoclip (with or without epinephrine preinjection), there was a significantly higher rate of residual DEP positive signal for underlying arterial blood flow in patients with major SRH than in intermediate SRH (27% vs 14%). None of the patients with oozing bleeding had a positive DEP signal after standard endoscopic hemostasis whereas 35% of those with spurting arterial bleeding (Forrest IA) still had residual arterial blood flow. Concerning clinical relevant outcomes, the 30-day rebleed rate was 29% in patients with spurting arterial bleeding (Forrest IA) ulcers and 0% in the oozing ulcer group.[7] Residual arterial blood flow after visually guided endoscopic hemostasis was highly correlated with ulcer rebleeding. In this cohort study, rebleeding occurred in 80% of patients who had residual arterial blood flow after visually guided hemostasis according to current standard of care recommendations for spurting ulcers treated endoscopically.

Results of a recent RCT evaluating DEP for NVUGI bleeding—including peptic ulcers, Dieulafoy lesions, and Mallory-Weiss tears—reported significantly higher 30-day rates of rebleeding in the standard therapy group compared with the DEP-assisted treatment

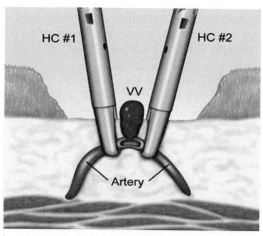

Fig. 3. Diagram of hemoclip (HC) placement next to a visible vessel (VV) in the ulcer base to occlude the underlying artery and obliteration blood flow and thereby prevent rebleeding.

group.[9] These findings confirm the importance of underlying arterial blood flow as a major risk factor for rebleeding of NVUGI bleeding. Specifically, as a risk factor, residual arterial blood flow underneath stigmata highly correlates with ulcer rebleeding. If more endoscopic treatment is successfully applied to obliterate underlying arterial blood flow, however, there is a significant improvement in clinical outcomes for patients with severe NVUGI hemorrhage. Confirming the RCT outcome results, the authors recently reported a multivariable regression analysis of a larger cohort of CURE hemostasis ulcer patients comparing those treated before DEP was available as historical controls with the current DEP RCT–treated patients. Patients treated with DEP guidance had significantly fewer rebleeds and surgeries[16] and also reduced mortality than matched historical control patients not treated with DEP. In contrast, RCT patients in the standard treatment group of the RCT (eg, treated with standard visually guided hemostasis) had no differences in clinical outcomes compared with matched historical controls.[16]

HEMOSTASIS: STANDARD TREATMENTS FOR NONVARICEAL GASTROINTESTINAL HEMORRHAGE
Fundamentals

The goals of endoscopic hemostasis are control of active bleeding and prevention of rebleeding by sealing the underlying artery.[17] This can usually be achieved by different techniques but the results are not always definitive—resulting in no rebleeds or adverse events.

Thermal Contact Probes

Heater probes, bipolar probes, and multipolar electrocoagulation (MPEC) probes have been the foundation of endoscopic hemostasis for many years.[10] Thermal probes lead to hemostasis by 2 mechanisms to result in coaptive coagulation: tamponade of the underlying artery to interrupt blood flow and application of enough thermal energy to seal the artery.[17] These probes are often effective for different types of nonvariceal bleeding lesions with major stigmata, including peptic ulcers, Mallory-Weiss tears, and Dieulafoy lesions. The authors recommend low-power settings for MPEC of NVGI lesions, ranging between 12 W and 15 W, with the duration of energy application and amount of pressure depending on the expected depth and size of the vessel being treated and the wall thickness of the gut.[8,10,17] In the laboratory, arteries up to approximately 2 mm in diameter could be coaptively closed with thermal probes at low-power settings by first applying firm tamponade to interrupt arterial blood flow and then by coagulating with up to 150 J before moving the probe. Larger thermal probes (10F size) coagulate larger, deeper arteries more effectively than smaller (7F size), because interruption of the underlying blood flow is more effective and the coagulation zone is bigger with the larger probes.[10,17] For larger vessels located underneath peptic ulcers, or Dieulafoy lesions, firm pressure and slow coagulation for 8 seconds to 10 seconds with several tamponade positions on either side of the SRH is usually sufficient for good hemostasis with these thermal probes.[10]

Thermal probes are also used to treat GI bleeding from vascular ectasias or small GI angiomas. Smaller, superficial vessels, such as vascular ectasias, can be treated with light pressure for 1 second to 2 seconds and a low-power setting of 12 W. The lower-power setting and tamponade pressure are appropriate for thinner-walled organs, such as the small intestine and right colon.

The main risk of using a thermal probe is perforation, with excessive application of coagulation or pressure, especially in acute or nonfibrotic lesions. Transmural injury and postcoagulation syndrome can also result in the colon. Thermal probes also cause coagulation injury, which can increase ulcer or lesion size and depth, which might increase the risk of delayed bleeding, particularly in patients with coagulopathies.[10,17–19]

Injection Therapy

This is performed with a sclerotherapy needle to inject epinephrine (diluted to a concentration of 1:10,000 or 1:20,000 in saline) submucosally into or around the bleeding site or in the ulcer base around the SRH. Typically, 3 to 4 injections, each 1 mL in volume, are injected around the SRH. Epinephrine alone can temporarily reduce arterial blood flow in ulcers with major stigmata by vasoconstriction, but blood flow often returns and rebleeding can result.[7] This technique is widely available and safe for use in patients. It is not as effective for definitive hemostasis, however, as thermal coagulation or endoscopic clips and is not recommended to be used alone. Instead, it is now recommended to combine epinephrine injection with either thermal or hemoclip hemostasis.[20–23]

Endoscopic Clips (Hemoclips)

Standard hemoclips are passed through the endoscope suction channel and can mechanically close the bleeding artery underlying the SRH vessel.[7,9,10] After DEP localization of the artery underlying the SRH in PUBs, the authors recommend hemoclipping on either side of the SRH to occlude the artery and provide definitive hemostasis[7,9,10] (see **Fig. 3**). This can be done with or without preinjection with epinephrine, which is usually used to prepare the field if active bleeding is evident. Hemoclips offer comparable efficacy to thermal probes in achieving definitive hemostasis.[24] By not causing thermal damage and enlargement of lesions, hemoclips are especially useful in patients with malnutrition, reduced healing, or coagulopathies. But they can be difficult or impossible to deploy because of lesion location (such as the posterior bulb of the duodenum) or a fibrotic ulcer base.

Over-the-Scope (Large) Hemoclip

A large over-the-scope clip is used for both salvage hemostasis for ulcers that rebleed and more recently for primary hemostasis of NVUGI bleeding lesions or large, fibrotic ulcers.[25] In a recent RCT, Schmidt and colleagues[26] reported significantly better outcomes with the over-the-scope clip compared with standard through-the-endoscope treatment of patients with PUB rebleeding. To explain why, when DEP was used to monitor arterial blood flow under SRH in PUBs in a prospective CURE study, patients treated with the over-the-scope clip had significantly lower residual arterial flows than those patients treated with standard hemostasis (MPEC coagulation or through-the-scope hemoclipping with or without epinephrine injection). The explanation seems to be that the over-the-scope clip is a larger, more powerful hemoclip that grasps more tissue and is capable of mechanically compressing and sealing larger, deeper arteries than standard hemostasis techniques (DM Jensen, personal communication, 2017). Particularly for large, fibrotic ulcers and anastomotic ulcers, such large powerful clips have the potential of significantly improving endoscopic hemostasis of NVUGI lesions, such as PUBs and Dieulafoy lesions.[27]

COLONIC DIVERTICULAR HEMORRHAGE AND THE DOPPLER ENDOSCOPIC PROBE

Over the past few decades, there has been increased utilization of urgent colonoscopy after colon purge for patients presenting with severe hematochezia from suspected colon sources. This is particularly useful for lesion localization, risk stratification, colonoscopic diagnosis, and hemostasis of focal colon lesions with SRH, including diverticulosis.[28–30] When the colon is cleared of stool, clots, and blood, major stigmata of recent diverticular hemorrhage can often be recognized and effectively treated by experienced endoscopists. In contrast, angiography does not usually provide an etiologic diagnosis nor identify nonbleeding SRH. Urgent colonoscopy after effective colonic purge offers a significant incremental improvement over angiography in diagnostic and therapeutic yield. That is because only active bleeding of high volume can be localized and effectively treated with angiography whereas urgent colonoscopy with a good colon preparation can identify both bleeding and nonbleeding SRH (such as adherent clots, visible vessels, or flat spots in colon diverticula) as well as mucosal lesions and other focal colonic lesions.[28–30]

The authors recently reported a prospective study of the natural history of definitive diverticular hemorrhage (defined as finding a major SRH in a diverticulum) and colonoscopic Doppler blood flow monitoring for risk stratification and as a guide to definitive hemostasis.[31] The study only included patients with severe diverticular bleeding who had SRH on colonoscopy. All patients were treated with medical treatment alone without colonoscopic hemostasis and the 30-day rebleeding rates were compared for low-risk SRH (flat spots or clean-based diverticula after clots washed away) versus high-risk SRH (active arterial bleeding, NBVV, or adherent clot). None of the patients with low-risk SRH had rebleeding on medical treatment, whereas 76% of patients with high-risk SRH rebled. In those patients studied with the DEP, 92% with high-risk SRH had superficial (<4 mm deep) arterial flow detected underneath and for 2 mm to 4 mm on either side of the SRH in the diverticulum. For endoscopic hemostasis details, for approximately 50% of patients with definitive diverticula hemorrhage, the SRH was found at the neck of the diverticulum and 50% at the base.[31] The location of the SRH in the diverticulum has been used as a guide to safe and effective colonoscopic hemostasis. For SRH in the base of the diverticulum, hemoclipping is recommended (**Fig. 4**). In contrast, if the SRH on the diverticulum is at the neck, MPEC probe with lateral coagulation is fast, effective, and safe for obliterating underlying arterial flow and prevent rebleeding (**Fig. 5**). Since colon DEP catheters have been available and used as guides to hemostasis along with the SRH location (at the neck or base of the diverticulum), none of the patients in a prospective cohort had recurrent diverticular hemorrhage.[31] The

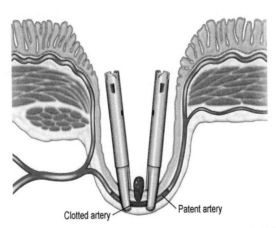

Clotted artery   Patent artery

Fig. 4. Diagram of hemoclipping the underlying artery next to an NBVV in a colonic. diverticulum base for definitive hemostasis. This is guided by DEP for localization of underlying arterial blood flow.

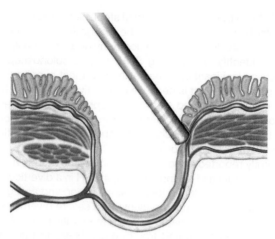

Fig. 5. Diagram of thermal coagulation with MPEC probe of a bleeding site at the neck of a colonic diverticulum. Checking for residual blood flow will confirm definitive hemostasis and help prevent rebleeding.

results from this study suggest that DEP-guided colonoscopic hemostasis can significantly reduce the rate of rebleeding in patients with colonic diverticular hemorrhage.

SUMMARY

Although standard endoscopic treatments are effective in providing definitive hemostasis for NVUGI bleeding lesions in many patients, there is room for significant improvement, particularly in high-risk patients. With major SRH, residual arterial blood flow is common after standard visually guided hemostasis. DEP has proved a valuable tool for risk stratification and as a guide to definitive hemostasis in such patients. If residual arterial blood flow is present, further treatment can be applied after initial visually guided initial hemostasis. A recent RCT and a multivariable regression analysis have reported that DEP-guided treatment is safe and improves clinical outcomes (rebleeding, surgery, and mortality) compared with standard hemostasis of NVUGI hemorrhage. Recent results suggest that DEP is valuable for risk stratification, for documenting complete hemostasis, and in improving clinical outcomes of both NVUGI hemorrhage and definitive diverticular hemorrhage. Monitoring of underlying arterial blood flow is now feasible with DEP. Residual arterial blood flow after endoscopic hemostasis is a major risk factor for rebleeding of nonvariceal GI lesions. Therefore, the authors highly recommended using DEP as a bedside guide during urgent endoscopy or colonoscopy to improve risk stratification and definitive endoscopic hemostasis.

REFERENCES

1. Abougergi MS, Travis AC, Saltzman JR. The in-hospital mortality rate for upper GI hemorrhage has decreased over 2 decades in the United States: a nationwide analysis. Gastrointest Endosc 2015;81:882–8.
2. Halland M, Young M, Fitzgerald MN, et al. Characteristics and outcomes of upper gastrointestinal hemorrhage in a tertiary referral hospital. Dig Dis Sci 2010;55: 3430–5.
3. Strate LL, Ayanian JZ, Kotler G, et al. Risk factors for mortality in lower intestinal bleeding. Clin Gastroenterol Hepatol 2008;6:1004–10.

4. Gralnek IM, Neeman Z, Strate LL. Acute lower GI bleeding. N Engl J Med 2017; 376:1054–63.

5. Laursen SB, Leontiades GL, Stanley AJ, et al. Relationship between timing of endoscopy and mortality with peptic ulcer bleeding: a nationwide cohort study. Gastrointest Endosc 2017;85:936–44.

6. Forrest JA, Finlayson ND, Shearman DJ. Endoscopy in gastrointestinal bleeding. Lancet 1974;2:394–7.

7. Jensen DM, Ohning GV, Kovacs TOG, et al. Doppler endoscopic probe as a guide to risk stratification and definitive hemostasis of peptic ulcer bleeding. Gastrointest Endosc 2016;83:129–36.

8. Barkun AN, Bardou M, Kuipers EJ, et al. International consensus recommendations on the management of patients with nonvariceal upper gastrointestinal bleeding. Ann Intern Med 2010;152:101–13.

9. Jensen DM, Kovacs TOG, Ohning GV, et al. Doppler endoscopic probe monitoring of blood flow improves risk stratitification and outcomes of patients with severe nonvariceal upper gastrointestinal hemorrhage. Gastroenterology 2017;152: 1310–8.

10. Jensen DM, Machicado GA. Endoscopic hemostasis of ulcer hemorrhage with injection, thermal, or combination methods. Tech Gastrointest Endosc 2005;7: 124–31.

11. Jensen DM, Eklund S, Persson T, et al. Reassessment of rebleeding risk of Forrest IB (oozing) peptic ulcer bleeding in a large international randomized trial. Am J Gastroenterol 2017;112:441–6.

12. Gralnek IM, Dumonceau JM, Kuipers EJ, et al. Diagnosis and management of nonvariceal upper gastrointestinal hemorrhage: European society of gastrointestinal endoscopy (ESGE) guideline. Endoscopy 2015;47:a1–46.

13. Beckly DE, Casebow MP, Pettengell KE. The use of a Doppler ultrasound probe for localizing arterial blood flow during upper gastrointestinal endoscopy. Endoscopy 1982;14:146–7.

14. Wong RC. Endoscopic Doppler US probe for acute peptic ulcer hemorrhage. Gastrointest Endosc 2004;60:804–12.

15. Wong RC, Chak A, Kobayashi K, et al. Role of Doppler US in acute peptic ulcer hemorrhage: can it predict failure of endoscopic therapy? Gastrointest Endosc 2000;52:315–21.

16. Jensen DM, Jensen ME, Markovic D, et al. Is hemostasis with Doppler endoscopic probe guidance an improvement compared to visually guided treatment of severe ulcer hemorrhage? Gastroenterol 2017;152:S474.

17. Johnston JH, Jensen DM, Auth D. Experimental comparison of endoscopic yttrium-aluminum-garnet laser, electrosurgery, and heater probe for canine gut arterial coagulation. Importance of compression and avoidance of erosion. Gastroenterology 1987;92:1101–8.

18. Jensen DM. Thermal probe or combination therapy for nonvariceal upper gastrointestinal hemorrhage. Tech Gastrointest Endosc 1999;1:107–14.

19. Laine L, Long GL, Bakos GJ, et al. Optimizing bipolar electrocoagulation for endoscopic hemostasis: assessment of factors influencing energy delivery and coagulation. Gastrointest Endosc 2008;67:502–8.

20. Barkun AN, Martel M, Toubouti Y, et al. Endoscopic hemostasis in peptic ulcer bleeding for patients with high-risk lesions: a series of meta-analyses. Gastrointest Endosc 2009;69:786–99.

21. Laine L, Jensen DM. Management of patients with ulcer bleeding. Am J Gastroenterol 2012;107:345–60.

22. Marmo R, Rotondano G, Piscopo R, et al. Dual therapy versus monotherapy in the endoscopic treatment of high-risk bleeding ulcers: a meta-analysis of controlled trials. Am J Gastroenterol 2007;102:279–89.

23. Vergara M, Bennett C, Calvet X, et al. Epinephrine injection versus epinephrine injection and a second endoscopic method in high-risk bleeding ulcers. Cochrane Database Syst Rev 2014;(10):CD005584.

24. Sung JJ, Tsoi KK, Lai LH, et al. Endoscopic clipping versus injection and thermocoagulation in the treatment of non-variceal upper gastrointestinal bleeding: a meta-analysis. Gut 2007;56:1364–73.

25. Wedi E, von Renteln D, Gonzalez S, et al. Use of the over-the-scope-clip (OTSC) in non-variceal upper gastrointestinal bleeding in patients with severe cardiovascular comorbidities: a retrospective study. Endosc Int Open 2017;5(9):E875–82.

26. Schmidt A, Goelder S, Messmann H, et al. Over-the-scope-clips versus standard endoscopic therapy in patients with recurrent peptic ulcer bleeding. Preliminary results of a prospective randomized multicenter trial ("STING"). United European Gastro J 2016;02(Suppl 01).

27. Chan SM, Lau JYW. Can we now recommend OTSC as first-line therapy in case of non-variceal upper gastrointestinal bleeding? Endosc Int Open 2017;05:E883–5.

28. Jensen DM, Machicado GA, Jutabha R, et al. Urgent colonoscopy for the diagnosis and treatment of severe diverticular hemorrhage. N Engl J Med 2000; 342:78–82.

29. Jensen DM, Machicado GA. Diagnosis and treatment of severe hematochezia—the role of urgent colonoscopy after purge. Gastroenterol 2009;137:1897–902.

30. Jensen DM, Machicado GA. Colonoscopy for the diagnosis and treatment of severe lower gastrointestinal bleeding; routine outcomes and cost analysis. Gastrointest Endosc Clin N Am 1997;7:77–98.

31. Jensen DM, Ohning GV, Kovacs TOG. Natural history of definitive diverticular hemorrhage based on stigmata of recent hemorrhage and colonoscopic Doppler blood flow monitoring for risk stratification and definitive hemostasis. Gastrointest Endosc 2016;83:416–23.

The Role of Transcatheter Arterial Embolization in the Management of Nonvariceal Upper Gastrointestinal Bleeding

Dan E. Orron, MD[a], Allan I. Bloom, MD, FSIR[b], Ziv Neeman, MD[c],*

KEYWORDS

- Arterial • Embolization • Embolic agents
- Nonvariceal upper gastrointestinal bleeding • Hemorrhage • Interventional radiology

KEY POINTS

- Current technology advances have introduced microcatheters that are capable of selecting third-order branches and of delivering a wide array of embolic agents.
- The majority of cases of nonvariceal upper gastrointestinal bleeding are managed conservatively or by endoscopy, which has also benefited from significant technological advances.
- With the advancement of endoscopic bleeding control hemostatic techniques, patients with nonvariceal upper gastrointestinal bleeding are generally referred to the interventional radiologist for therapeutic management.
- This paper reviews the clinical, technical, and angiographic variables that guide appropriate embolization strategies aiming to optimize the anticipated outcome of transcatheter arterial embolization.

INTRODUCTION

The usefulness of diagnostic angiography in localizing GI hemorrhage was described by Margulis and colleagues[1] and Baum and associates[2] in the 1960s. Before this breakthrough, barium studies of the gastrointestinal (GI) tract were the only imaging adjunct to plain abdominal radiography. Transcatheter infusion of the constricting agent vasopressin was the first endovascular means of hemostasis applied to GI bleeding (GIB),[3,4] after which transcatheter arterial embolization (TAE), as it was described initially, using autologous blood clot.[5] In the ensuing years, continued innovation and technological advancements have resulted in TAE becoming an effective

Disclosure Statement: No disclosures for all 3 authors.
[a] Department of Radiology, Carmel Medical Center, Michal Street, Haifa 34362, Israel; [b] Department of Radiology, Hadassah University Medical Center, Ein Karem, Jerusalem 91120, Israel; [c] Medical Imaging Institute, Haemek Medical Center, Izhak Rabin Boulevard, Afula 1834111, Israel
* Corresponding author.
E-mail address: ziv_ne@clalit.org.il

Gastrointest Endoscopy Clin N Am 28 (2018) 331–349
https://doi.org/10.1016/j.giec.2018.02.006
1052-5157/18/© 2018 Elsevier Inc. All rights reserved.

and rapid means of achieving hemostasis, particularly in hemodynamically unstable patients with acute, massive nonvariceal upper GIB (NVUGIB) that could not be accessed or controlled endoscopically. Angiography is also used to identify and treat causes of chronic bleeding in which endoscopy failed to identify a source.

IMAGING DIAGNOSIS OF GASTROINTESTINAL BLEEDING

Before the development of multidetector computed tomography (MDCT) scanning techniques, radionuclide scanning with tagged red blood cells/sulfur colloid was the primary noninvasive imaging modality for detection and localization of GIB, owing to its high sensitivity. Scintigraphy can detect bleeding rates as low as 0.1 mL/s, whereas angiographic detection requires a bleeding rate of 0.5 to 1.0 mL/s.[6–11]

Nuclear scanning is useful for differentiating between upper and lower GIB (LGIB) and detecting multiple sites of bleeding, although it provides no etiologic information. Limitations in UGIB include activity in the heart, lung and spleen, secretion of free technetium pertechnate into the stomach and antegrade movement of the tracer from the stomach to bowel owing to peristalsis. In current practice, radionuclide scanning has occasional usefulness in LGIB but no role in UGIB.

MDCT has largely replaced radionuclide scanning for the assessment of LGIB in stable patients, and has demonstrated a bleeding rate sensitivity intermediate to that of isotope scanning and catheter angiography. In an animal model reported by Kuhle and Sheiman,[10] bleeding rates as low as 0.3 mL/min were identified. Current imaging technology allows the demonstration of small bleeding arteries. Best results are obtained with the triphasic technique (precontrast, arterial, and portal phases). MDCT is most suitable to, and has been most studied in, acute LGIB.[11–15] The overall sensitivity and specificity have been reported at 79% to 89% and 85% to 95%, respectively.[11,16,17] Importantly, for the scenarios in which endoscopy either did not identify a bleed, or identified a bleed but could not determine the source, the American College of Radiology considers MDCT to be a diagnostic modality equivalent to angiography.[18] For cases in which a small bowel bleeding source is suspected, the addition of neutral (water density) oral contrast agent (CT enterography) improves the detection of small bowel pathology.

CT is also useful for detecting related pathology such as tumors and aneurysms/pseudoaneurysms. Treatment planning (access and catheter selection) is facilitated by its demonstration of relevant anatomy, particularly patency/tortuosity of the access arteries and presence of aortic visceral branch anomalies or origin narrowing/angulation.

Cone beam CT, a standard feature in current angiographic units, allows catheterization guidance by overlay of the CT angiography image upon live fluoroscopy (fusion road map). In addition, Cone beam CT is superior to digital subtraction angiography for detection of residual untreated tumor after embolization.[19]

MDCT is rarely required for the assessment of NVUGIB, except in rare cases in which endoscopy cannot be performed completely. Exceptions include patients with a history of pancreatitis, and recent percutaneous or endoscopic biliary procedures. MDCT may also be useful in patients with concomitant portal hypertension.

DIAGNOSTIC ANGIOGRAPHY

In current practice, patients with NVUGIB are referred for angiography with a therapeutic rather than a diagnostic intention. The typical patient is hemodynamically unstable with massive bleeding resistant to medical management and endoscopic intervention. Less common indications include failure to identify a bleeding source by endoscopy or CT, chronic bleeding, and postoperative hemorrhage. Preprocedural assessment includes review of patient history, laboratory results, endoscopic and imaging findings, and pulses at possible access sites. Coagulopathy and renal insufficiency/failure are corrected if possible. It is important to remember that angiography and transarterial embolization (TAE) are part of the resuscitative process. Infusions and blood products can be given during the procedure, and therefore excessive delays are unnecessary. A longer interval between the onset of bleeding and the time of TAE has been correlated to a greater early rebleed rate.[20]

An additional benefit of MDCT, particularly in the elderly, is the information provided for planning of the angiographic procedure, particularly with regard to the presence of vascular occlusive disease and tortuosity along planned access route (femoral or upper extremity), patency, and severe caudad angulation of the visceral branch origins. This information may alert the operator to choose an upper extremity (brachial or radial) approach over the femoral approach. Informed consent is then obtained after an explanation of the procedure, alternative options, benefits, and risks.

The presence of bloody return on gastric lavage after the evacuation of clots correlates with a greater likelihood of the angiogram being positive. This differs from LGIB in which bloody stools may occur after bleeding cessation. For cases of NVUGIB in which the bleeding site has been identified by endoscopy or imaging, the procedure should begin with selective angiograms of the celiac and left gastric arteries. Abdominal aortography is not routinely performed except for instances of difficult anatomy, because it involves a large contrast dose and usually does not demonstrate the bleeding source, which commonly arises from third-order branches.[21] Patients with bleeding duodenal ulcers may on occasion present with rectal bleeding with negative lavage, owing to competence of the pylorus. In these instances, the superior mesenteric artery (SMA) and the inferior mesenteric artery are studied as well to exclude a lower GI source.[11]

Preshaped catheters commonly used for catheterization of the celiac artery and SMA include the 4F to 5F Cobra (Cook Medical), Mikaelson (Merit, South Jordan, UT), Omni SOS (AngioDynamics, Latham, NY), and sidewinder catheters. A Waltmans loop may be required to select the left gastric artery (LGA). If there are no signs of bleeding on angiogram from the main vessel origin, superselective angiography of each possible blood supply is performed using a microcatheter placed through the diagnostic catheter (coaxial technique). Prolonged injection time and use of carbon dioxide as a contrast agent increase the detection of small hemorrhagic foci.[22]

Tortuosity of the parent or branch vessel, and steeply angled origin or osteal narrowing of the branch vessel may render superselective catheterization of arterial branches such as the inferior phrenic and left gastric difficult.[23] Available maneuvers for overcoming these difficulties include creating a cleft in the tip of the diagnostic catheter so that the microcatheter is directed toward the angulation,[24] the turn back technique,[25] preshaping the microwire into a Shepard's hook form,[26] and the balloon blocking technique.[27]

The angiographer must be aware of the vascular arcades supplying each segment of the upper GI tract,[11] because TAE must account for the possibility of retrograde flow to the bleeding site after embolization of 1 side of the arcade.

The esophageal supply involves a network of intercommunicating arteries and several discrete supplying arteries.[28] The proximal esophagus is supplied by the inferior thyroid branch of the thyrocervical trunk. The midportion of the esophagus is supplied by multiple thoracic aortic branches including the bronchial arteries. The distal esophagus is supplied by the LGA and ascending branches of the left phrenic artery.

The arcade supplying the lesser curvature of the stomach is formed by the LGA and the right gastric artery branch off the left hepatic artery. The greater curvature of the stomach is supplied by the gastroepiploic arcade formed by the right gastroepiploic branch of the gastroduodenal artery (GDA) and the left gastroepiploic branch of the splenic artery. This arcade is complete in approximately two-thirds of patients.[22]

Gastric hemorrhage most commonly involves the LGA (85%), followed by the right gastric artery (5%), short gastric 5%, gastroepiploic (3%), phrenic (1%), and gastroduodenal arteries (1%).[29]

The GDA provides dominant supply to the duodenum and forms the pancreaticoduodenal arcade with the inferior pancreaticoduodenal (IPDA) branch of the SMA. The 3 major branches of the GDA are the supraduodenal, posterior superior, and anterior superior pancreaticoduodenal arteries, beyond which the artery continues as the right gastroepiploic artery. Commonly, both the GDA and IPDA supply the hemorrhage.

VARIANTS

A description of the types and frequencies of anatomic variants regarding the upper GI arterial supply is beyond the scope of this article and has been described elsewhere.[30,31] The celiac artery arises anteriorly as the first major branch of the abdominal aorta, usually at the level of the T12 to L1 intervertebral space. In most instances it measures 1.5 to 2.8 cm in length and divides into the left gastric, splenic, and common hepatic arteries. Variants occur in 10% to 15% of cases, the most common are the gastrosplenic trunk and hepatosplenic trunks.[31]

The LGA may alternately arise from the splenic artery or directly from the aorta. The right gastric artery most commonly arises from the proper hepatic (50%) or left hepatic arteries (15%), but may also arise from the middle hepatic, GDA, right hepatic artery, or common hepatic arteries.

The GDA usually arises from the proper hepatic artery, but may also arise from the right hepatic artery, including the right hepatic artery replaced to the SMA or from the celiac trunk.[22] The supraduodenal artery is present in 93% of cases and supplies the distal two-thirds of the upper duodenum. Its possible origins include the GDA (27%), common hepatic (20%), left hepatic (20%), and right hepatic arteries (13%).

Common variants relating to hepatic supply include replaced or accessory right hepatic artery from the SMA, replaced left hepatic artery from the LGA, and SMA origin of the common hepatic artery.

Angiographic Findings

Identification of the bleeding artery is the initial step. The cardinal angiographic finding in active hemorrhage is contrast extravasation into the bowel lumen at the bleeding site (**Figs. 1** and **2**). Active extravasation appears as an amorphous extraluminal contrast collection not conforming to a tubular shape, which may enter and opacify the bowel lumen. The presence of extravasated contrast within bowel folds (the pseudovein sign), is differentiated from a vein by its persistence beyond the venous phase. Artifacts resulting from peristalsis and normal adrenal gland blush can be identified by careful comparison of subtracted and nonsubtracted images.[21] Hyperemia commonly produces a mucosal blush. Extravasation or mucosal blush were identified in 61% of cases referred owing to UGIB.[32] The likelihood of extravasation is greater in the presence of hemodynamic instability and significant blood transfusion requirements.[33]

Owing to the intermittent nature of GIB, no angiographic abnormalities may be identified, particularly regarding bleeding from peptic ulcer. Occlusion or sharp angulation of a branch may imply the presence of recent bleeding. In such cases, superselective catheterization and contrast injection may dislodge a clot and allow for the demonstration of extravasation, and for TAE.[11] Additional secondary angiographic signs suggestive of a bleeding source in the absence of extravasation include hyperemia,

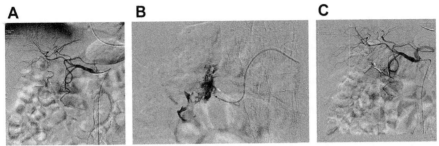

Fig. 1. Transarterial embolization of a gastroduodenal artery bleed after failed endoscopic clipping. (*A*) Common hepatic arteriogram demonstrates contrast extravasation from a branch of the gastroduodenal artery (*arrow*). The curved arrow marks an endoscopically placed coil. (*B*) Superselective angiogram of the bleeding branch via microcatheter reveals extravasation and opacification of duodenal lumen (*arrow*). (*C*) Common hepatic angiogram after coil embolization demonstrates occlusion of the bleeding branch, absence of extravasation, and maintained patency of the gastroduodenal artery. Arrow points to the Endoclip.

pseudoaneurysm, arteriovenous fistula, or prominent early draining vein. Mass lesions are identified by the presence of tumor vascularity, mass effect (draping, displacement), or encasement/narrowing of regional arteries. Calcification may indicate the presence of an aneurysm.

The introduction of digital subtraction angiography has significantly reduced procedure time and contrast dose. Although the contrast sensitivity of digital subtraction angiography is greater than that of conventional (cut film) angiography, the overall resolution is inferior, and the technique is limited by patient motion and peristalsis. The latter may be reduced by the intravenous administration of 1 mg glucagon. For intubated patients, cessation of respiration during image acquisition is useful.

Standard software guidance techniques (road map) allow real-time guidance for vessel catheterization by overlaying the angiographic image with live fluoroscopy, or, as mentioned, with a CT angiography image (fusion road map).

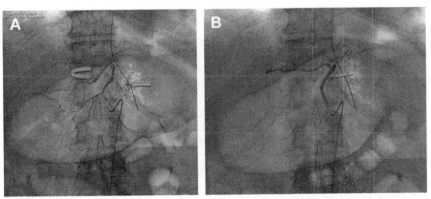

Fig. 2. Transarterial embolization of an active gastric bleed owing to erosive disease. (*A*) Selective left gastric artery angiogram demonstrates contrast extravasation in the proximal stomach (*thick arrow*). Note variant origin of the left hepatic artery from the left gastric artery (*curved arrow*). (*B*) Left gastric artery angiogram after coiling of the bleeding branch (*arrow*) demonstrates absence of extravasation, occlusion of the bleeding branch, and maintained patency of the left gastric artery and left hepatic artery.

Empiric embolization may be considered when a bleeding site was localized by endoscopy but could not be controlled, and no extravasation is identified upon selective angiography.[20,34] The clinical outcome of empiric embolization is similar to that of nonempiric embolization.[11,35–38] Endoscopic placement of a hemoclip at the bleeding site is a useful localizing aid. Critically ill patients with hypovolemia are prone to vasoconstriction, which can cause an absence of extravasation on selective angiograms. Upon correction of hypovolemia and vasoconstriction, the artery may expand resulting in rebleeding. Any coils placed earlier may migrate distally to the point of a new caliber match,[38] possibly allowing rebleed.

PROVOCATIVE ANGIOGRAPHY AND LOCALIZATION MANEUVERS

Arterial GI hemorrhages are frequently intermittent and not present at the time of selective angiography. In hemodynamically stable patients, particularly for cases of chronic, intermittent LGIB, provocative transcatheter injection of a vasodilator (verapamil 100–200 µg or nitroglycerin 100–300 µg), anticoagulant (heparin 3000–10,000 U), or a thrombolytic agent (tissue plasminogen activator, 5–10 mg) may reactivate bleeding and improve detection from 32% to 69%.[39–42] The yield of this maneuver is greater in patients with prior episodes of massive bleeding.

Blood products should be available in case bleeding is reactivated and not controllable by endovascular means. In the event a small bowel lesion is identified, its location may be marked for the surgeon by the placement of a microcoil or leaving a microcatheter and injecting methylene blue.[11,43–45] Although there seems to be a role for provocative angiography in recurrent NVUGIB, prospective trials are lacking.[22]

CAUSES OF NONVARICEAL UPPER GASTROINTESTINAL BLEEDING

Erosive entities account for the majority of NVUGIB. Less common causes include Mallory-Weiss tears, angiodysplasias, neoplasms, and aortoenteric fistula. The typical angiographic finding in Mallory-Weiss tears upon selective LGA or inferior phrenic arteriogram is linear contrast collections in the vicinity of the gastroesophageal junction.

Angiodysplasia, or angioectasias, are an acquired degenerative arteriovenous pathology associated with hemorrhage, which is typically chronic, recurrent, and self-limited. This entity accounts for 5% to 10% of acute UGIB and may present with a wide range of severity. Isolated ectasias differ endoscopically from the diffuse ectasias found in gastric antral vascular ectasia, also referred to as "watermelon stomach."[22,46] an entity thought to be distinct from portal hypertensive gastropathy. Although most commonly found in elderly patients in the small bowel and colon, angiodysplasia can involve the stomach and duodenum.[47] The typical angiographic features include a tangle of vessels with early, prolonged and prominent filling of the draining vein (**Fig. 3**). Concomitant opacification of the artery and vein during an angiographic series is the basis for the typical tram track sign. TAE can be therapeutic in the face of failed endoscopy.[48]

The Dieulafoy lesion (**Fig. 4**), which accounts for less than 5% of acute UGIB, represents an aberrantly prominent (1–5 mm) arteriole, known as a "caliber-persistent artery," which produces hemorrhage by erosion of the submucosa, most commonly located below the gastroesophageal junction. TAE is an effective modality when endoscopic management fails, although the presence of multiple feeding vessels may limit success.[49]

Neoplasms also account for less than 5% of all UGIB.[50] Tumor-related bleeding beyond the ampulla of Vater is difficult to control endoscopically owing to blood

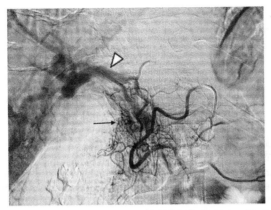

Fig. 3. Duodenal vascular malformation. Gastroduodenal artery angiogram demonstrates a tangle of vessels in the duodenum (*arrow*) and early, prominent opacification of the portal vein (*arrowhead*). (*Courtesy of* Ducksoo Kim MD, Boston University Medical Center, Boston MA; with permission.)

interference, and angiography may be required. Angiographic findings include vascular displacement, encasement, or narrowing by the mass, various degrees of tumor vascularity, and contrast extravasation (**Fig. 5**). TAE can provide a viable bridge to surgery if endoscopy fails or cannot reach the lesion.[51]

TAE is useful for the control of iatrogenic UGIB resulting from endoscopic sphincterotomy, which usually involves injury to the posterior pancreaticoduodenal branch of the GDA.[18] TAE is also useful for hemorrhage relating to percutaneous biliary drainage (**Fig. 6**), gastrostomy insertion, mycotic aneurysm (**Fig. 7**), pseudoaneurysm, and postoperative hemorrhage in which endoscopy is contraindicated.[18]

Aortoenteric fistula is a rare cause of NVUGIB resulting from communication between the aorta and the bowel. Diagnosis is made by endoscopy and/or CT. A pseudoaneurysm is usually identified at the site of fistula. Primary aortoenteric fistula usually involves the erosion of an abdominal aortic aneurysm into the distal duodenum. Historically, syphilis and tuberculous aortitis were common causes.[21] Secondary aortoenteric fistula occurs after reconstructive aortic surgery, usually in the vicinity of the proximal anastomosis. Surgical repair may be open or endovascular.

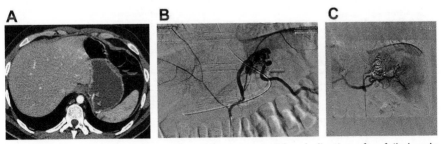

Fig. 4. Dieulafoy lesion in patient referred for transarterial embolization after failed endoscopic clipping. (*A*) Axial computed tomographic arteriography image at the level of the gastric fundus demonstrates prominent submucosal vessel in the posteromedial wall of the gastric fundus (*arrowheads*). (*B*) Midarterial image from a selective left gastric artery arteriogram reveals fundal tangle of vessels. Arrow indicates endoscopic clips. (*C*) Late arterial phase image of celiac angiogram after coil embolization demonstrating occlusion of the lesion.

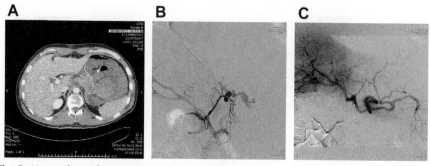

Fig. 5. Hemorrhage from gastric lymphoma managed by transarterial embolization (TAE). (*A*) Axial image of enhanced computed tomography at level of gastric fundus demonstrates enhancing soft tissue mass (*arrows*). (*B*) Midarterial phase image of the left gastric artery angiogram demonstrates pseudoaneurysm (*arrows*) and extravasation (*arrowhead*) arising from a branch of the left gastric artery. (*C*) Celiac angiogram after TAE with coils demonstrates absence of filling of the left gastric artery and pseudoaneurysms.

Endoscopic hemostasis may temporize the bleeding, although resection of the involved bowel is usually required.[21] Mortality in untreated cases has been reported to be as high as 100%.[21]

ENDOVASCULAR MANAGEMENT
Vasopressin Infusion

The intraarterial infusion of the octapeptide vasopressin (antidiuretic hormone), a vasoconstrictor of bowel arterioles and smooth muscle produced by the neurohypophysis, has long been applied to upper (Mallory-Weiss tears, erosive gastritis, stress ulcers[52–55]) and lower (colonic diverticulitis, angiodysplasia) GIB, with a reported success rate of 60% to 90%.[40,56] The treatment is less effective for duodenal bleeding,[57] owing to the dual blood supply, erosion of arteries too large to respond to

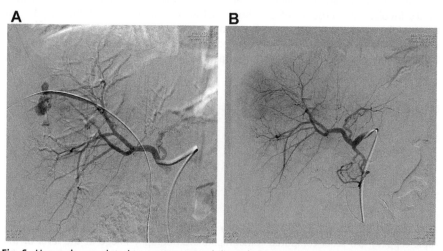

Fig. 6. Hemorrhage related to percutaneous biliary drainage managed by transarterial embolization. (*A*) Right hepatic arteriogram reveals extravasation (*arrowhead*) along the right PTC (percutaneous transhepatic cholangiography) tract. (*B*) after coil embolization of the culprit artery (*arrowheads*), there is no evidence of contrast extravasation.

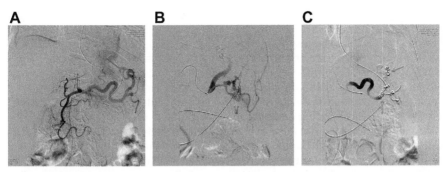

Fig. 7. Upper gastrointestinal bleed owing to mycotic aneurysm in the distal splenic artery resulting from giant gastric ulcer. (*A*) Celiac arteriogram demonstrates aneurysm in distal splenic artery (*arrowhead*). (*B*) Superselective splenic arteriogram identifies extravasation site (*arrow*). (*C*) Splenic arteriogram after coil embolization. There is no opacification of the distal splenic artery or pseudoaneurysm. Arrows represent coils.

vasopressin, and limitation of vessel constriction owing to chronic inflammatory changes or previous endoscopic electrocoagulation.

Vasopressin infusion is contraindicated in patients with coronary artery disease, severe hypertension, limb ischemia, and arrhythmias. The protocol[11] requires admission to intensive care and titrated administration of the agent into a catheter placed selectively into the bleeding artery. Recurrence of bleeding occurs in as many as 40% of patients, possibly owing to the inability of the agent to reach all potential collateral blood supply.[22] Adverse events are significant, including systemic (water retention, hyponatremia, hypertension), cardiovascular (myocardial ischemia, reduced cardiac output, arrhythmias, peripheral ischemia), and GI (cramping).[11] Acrocyanosis induced gangrene of the digits and penis has also been reported.[57] Dosages of vasopressin of more than 0.4 U/h are associated with a risk of bowel infarction and mesenteric–portal thrombosis.

In current practice, TAE has largely replaced vasopressin infusion, which may be considered for the management of active NVUGIB involving a branch that cannot be selectively catheterized, or when multiple bleeding points are noted to arise from a single artery.[11]

Transcatheter Embolization

TAE involves the placement, through an angiographic catheter, of an occlusive agent into the bleeding vessel, with the goal of inducing stasis-induced thrombosis while preserving collateral blood supply to avoid end-organ ischemia.[58] The development and continued improvement in coaxial catheter systems and embolic agents has allowed increasingly precise embolotherapy to achieve these goals.[21]

Upon selection of the bleeding artery, a 4F to 5F diagnostic catheter is positioned into the parent artery and a microcatheter (2.0–2.7F) is advanced through this catheter in a coaxial manner over a steerable, flexible, and shapeable microwire (0.014–0.018 inch) to the location of the bleed. Wire and catheter advancement are performed carefully under fluoroscopic guidance to minimize dissection and perforation. Vascular spasm is managed by the intraarterial administration of vasodilators (nitroglycerin 100–300 μg, or verapamil 100–200 μg).[21]

Embolic Agents

Postembolization thrombosis of the treated vessel results from promotion of 1 or more of the elements of Virchow's' triad—namely, stasis, endothelial injury, and hypercoagulability. The initial agent used to control GIB was autologous blood clot.[5]

Embolic agents may be divided into categories of temporary or permanent, and by type of agent (**Table 1**).

Hemostasis should be achieved safely and as quickly as possible. Choice of embolic material depends on the therapeutic goal of the procedure, and no single embolic agent is appropriate for every case; a combination of agents is commonly required. In addition to the duration of occlusion required, one must consider the size, elasticity, and flow of the target vessel, attainable catheter position and stability, and potential collateral filling of the bleeding vessel.[59]

The risk of bowel ischemia as an adverse event associated with TAE in the upper GI tract is considerably less than that of the lower GI vasculature owing to the presence of the arcades as described, and can be minimized by embolization as close to the bleeding site as possible. Patients with prior radiation therapy or surgical resection with arcade disruption are at increased risk of ischemia and in such cases a surgeon should be consulted before performing TAE.

Temporizing agents

Autologous blood clot was the initial agent used for TAE. This provides occlusion of 14 days' duration, but has been largely replaced by Gelfoam.

Gelfoam Absorbable gelatin sponge (Gelfoam, Pfizer, New York, NY) is a water-soluble biodegradable compressed gelatin made of purified porcine skin that functions as a sponge, absorbing up to 45 times its own weight in whole blood. In doing so, the injected Gelfoam swells, mechanically slows blood flow, and acts as a matrix for thrombus formation. The resulting occlusion is temporary (1–3 weeks), as preferred for hemostasis related to large vessels in benign disease and trauma. The Gelfoam can be administered in pledgelets, or as a slurry, which can be injected through a micro-catheter. When used alone for GIB, Gelfoam is associated with a higher early rebleed rate and, therefore, other agents should be deployed as well.[60,61] Gelfoam is also frequently used in conjunction with coils or plugs (sandwich technique) to achieve permanent occlusion, particularly in vascular beds where coils or plugs alone may not be adequate owing to collateral circulation. Gelfoam powder is not recommended for use in NVUGIB owing to variability of particle size, which may be as small as 50 μm, presenting a significant risk of bowel ischemia.[11,62]

Microfibrillar Bovine Collagen

Microfibrillar bovine collagen (Avitene, CR Bard, Inc., Murray Hill, NJ) is similar to Gelfoam, but provides a longer time to recanalization (partial in 2 weeks, complete in 2–3 months) as it promotes a granulomatous reaction.

Table 1
Embolic agents in use for upper gastrointestinal bleeding

Temporary	Autologous blood clot, Gelfoam (absorbable gelatin sponge), microfibrillar bovine collagen, thrombin, biodegradable starch microspheres.
Permanent	
Coils	Pushable, injectable, detachable (mechanical electric, hydrolytic).
Large vessel occluders	Vascular plugs (Amplatzer, MVP, GGVOD), Detachable balloons
Particles	Microspheres, polyvinyl alcohol.
Liquid agents	N-Butyl-2-cyanoacrylate glue (Glubran, GEM, Viareggio, Italy), Ethylene-vinyl alcohol copolymer (Onyx, Micro Therapeutics, Inc., Irvine, CA, USA).

Abbreviations: GGVOD, Gianturco-Grifka vascular occlusive device; MVP, microvascular plug.

Degradable Starch Microspheres (EmboCept)

EmboCept (PharmaCept GmbH, Berlin, Germany) is a deformable, starch microsphere of 50 μm diameter that is degraded by endogenous alpha-amylase into water soluble glucose molecules. The half-life is 35 minutes, and time to complete degradation is 2 hours.[59] The agent may have a role in tumor chemoembolization by allowing repeat embolization at short intervals and possibly reducing neoangiogenesis.[63,64]

Thrombin

Thrombin induces a hypercoagulable environment by cleaving soluble fibrinogen into fibrin, which eventually forms a cross-linked fibrin clot. The agent is not commonly used for UGIB, but may be considered as an adjunct to TAE or percutaneous occlusion of a large pseudoaneurysm.

Permanent Agents

Coils and plugs

These commonly used agents made of platinum, nitinol, stainless steel, or other alloys promote clotting by mechanical slowing of flow, and may contain prothrombotic material on the metallic skeleton. Coils are available in a wide range of shapes, diameters, and lengths, and may be delivered via a microcatheter or diagnostic catheter. The chosen diameter is usually 20% to 30% larger than the vessel diameter. An oversized coil may push the delivery catheter out of the vessel during deployment, resulting in nontarget embolization, whereas a coil too small will lodge distally to the target. Pushable coils are delivered by a wire or syringe injection. The injection force must be carefully controlled to avoid catheter displacement and nontarget embolization. Detachable and retrievable coils allow a more precise positioning and reduced risk of nontarget embolization. Plugs allow for controlled occlusion of larger arteries. These include the detachable Amplatzer Vascular Plug (Amplatzer Vascular Plug, AGA Medical Corporation, Plymouth, MN), POD (Penumbra, Alameda, CA), Medtronic Micro Vascular Plug (MVP; Medtronic, Minneapolis, MN), and the Azur Cx (Terumo Corporation, Tokyo, Japan). Coils and plugs provide mechanical obstruction analogous to placement of a surgical ligature.[40] Endothelial denudement and spasm induced by angiographic manipulation and deployed coils may facilitate thrombosis. However, in the presence of coagulopathy, this obstruction may not be adequate to achieve thrombosis and an additional agent is commonly required. Coils should be placed on either side (upstream and downstream) of the bleeding point. If intermediate sized arteries that cannot be catheterized are involved, the sandwich technique may be used, in which coils are placed on either side of the bleeding artery and Gelfoam or particles in between. Coil blockade may also be used to protect branches of the artery to be embolized from nontarget embolization. The deployment of a coil into the proximal aspect of the branch will prevent passage of particles to its vascular territory.

Particles

Embolic particles are made of inert synthetic materials such as polyvinyl alcohol and acrylic. The hemostatic mechanism resembles that of Gelfoam and collagen in the creation of a mechanical obstruction and provision of a matrix for thrombus formation. Particle size ranges from 75 to 1200 μm, enabling occlusion of a wide range of vessel sizes. The particles are mixed with contrast and injected until stasis is achieved, generally via a microcatheter. Injection is performed carefully in small boluses under fluoroscopic guidance, and the injection force is gradually reduced as angiographic forward progress is reduced and back flow is apparent. Particles are deployed when a "flow-directed strategy"[22] is indicated, as in the case of vascular tumors.

The catheter tip position must be distal to any major vascular branches. Use of particles 500 μ or greater is recommended to reduce risks of ischemia. The presence of arteriovenous shunting on the pretreatment angiogram is a contraindication to the use of particles unless coil blockade is feasible.

Liquid agents

This category includes the adhesive N-butyl cyanoacrylate (NBCA) and the nonadhesive ethylene-vinyl copolymer Onyx, which are particularly useful in occluding very small vascular branches. After superselective delivery via a microcatheter, these agents solidify and fill the vascular lumen mechanically so that thrombosis formation will occur regardless of whether coagulopathy is present (**Fig. 8**). NBCA is reported to significantly reduce procedure time in TAE for GIB and has a particular value in cases of massive hemorrhage in hemodynamically unstable and coagulopathic patients.[22,65] The polymerization rate of the glue upon contact with blood depends on the degree of its dilution with the fat-soluble contrast agent lipiodol. Overdilution will result in polymerization distal to the intended target; this is avoided by judicious technique and distal coil blockade. Underdilution may result in polymerization within the catheter and possibly adhesion of the catheter tip to the vessel wall. This is avoided by rapid removal of the microcatheter and aspiration of the guiding catheter.

Onyx has recently been introduced as an alternative to NBCA. Deployment is more easily controlled and has been applied to TAE for GIB with high success and negligible adverse events rates.[66,67] The drawback to use of Onyx is its high cost.

Strategies for transcatheter arterial embolization

Management of a bleed arising directly from the GDA is achieved by placing coils in the proximal GDA above and in the distal GDA below the point of extravasation. The intervening segment may be treated with Gelfoam pledgets (sandwich technique). Coil placement only above the point of extravasation will not be effective unless the IPDA (backdoor) is selected for placement of an additional coil distal to the bleed. Coils are quick and easy to deploy, and their deployment in the upper GI tract carries a very low risk of ischemia. Detachable and retrievable coils are useful to reduce the risk of nontarget embolization, particularly in the vicinity of key branch

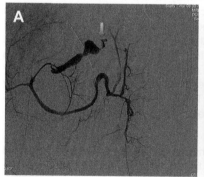
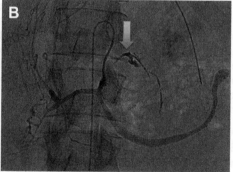

Fig. 8. Tumor hemorrhage from gastric tumor managed by transarterial embolization with cyanoacrylate. (*A*) Celiac angiogram demonstrates elongated pseudoaneurysm arising from the left gastric artery with a focus of extravasation at its distal end (*arrow*). (*B*) Postembolization celiac angiogram demonstrates occlusion of the pseudoaneurysm and no extravasation. The injected embolic material (*arrow*) is rendered opaque by the addition of the contrast agent lipiodol. (*Courtesy of* Gali Rozen MD, Tel Aviv Sourasky Medical Center, Tel Aviv, Israel; with permission.)

points. nontarget embolization of a coil to the hepatic artery is usually insignificant other than in the presence of portal hypertension, where it may produce catastrophic sequelae. Limitations of coils include limited ability to induce thrombosis in the coagulopathic patient and inability to reaccess the artery if rebleeding occurs. Therefore, an additional or alternate agent should be considered in the coagulopathic patient.[22] If the bleeding is from a branch that can be selected, such as the supraduodenal artery, hemostasis may be achieved by the deployment of microcoils, glue, or Onyx. The sandwich technique may be used if the vessel cannot be selected. The use of particles is generally reserved for bleeding from tumors.

Onyx and glue also are useful in cases where the bleeding artery was selected but the microcatheter cannot be advanced close to the artery. An example would be a fundal bleed supplied by the LGA. Another indication for these agents is hemorrhage from esophageal malignancy.[68]

Angiodysplasia and arteriovenous malformations may initially respond to embolization, but recurrent hemorrhage is frequent and resection is commonly required. The placement of a microcoil facilitates surgical localization.

Pseudoaneurysms of small vessels (4–5 mm) are managed by the occlusion of all feeding and draining arteries. Pseudoaneurysms of larger vessels may be managed by covered stent placement or coil embolization. Small articulate embolics are used to occlude the capillary bed of tumors, along with the liquid adhesive agents such as cyanoacrylate glue and Onyx.

RESULTS

Successful initial control of bleeding after TAE for NVUGIB has been reported in the range of 80% to 98% of patients.[22,69–72] Rebleeding can occur in up to 47% of patients, most commonly as the result of coagulopathy, the need to embolize in more than 1 vascular territory,[71] and in tumor-related bleeding.[72] Tumor-related bleeding limits clinical success owing to direct invasion of vascular structures and the development of chemotherapy or radiation therapy–induced mucositis.[72–75]

Loffroy and colleagues[22] recently reviewed 819 patients treated by TAE for acute NVUGIB. In almost all cases endoscopy had failed and the majority of patients were high-risk operative candidates. Clinical success ranged between 44% and 94%, with a rebleeding rate of 9% to 66%, and requirement for surgery of 2% to 35%; the adverse event rate was 0% to 26%. Overall, the 30-day mortality was 28%. Causes of technical failure included difficult anatomy, vascular dissection, spasm, multiple bleeding sites, and bleeding from tumors. One-half of the patients who rebled responded to a second TAE procedure.

COMPARISON WITH SURGERY

Operative management of NVUGIB is associated with a mortality of 10% to 30%.[76] A lack of comparative studies between TAE and surgery has long been noted.[32] Beggs and associates[76] recently performed a metaanalysis of 9 comparative studies involving 711 patients. The groups differed only by a greater incidence of ischemic heart disease and coagulopathy in the TAE groups. Rebleeding rates were greater in the TAE group, but if the oldest publications were removed, the difference was reduced. Retrograde filling of the bleeding site, a higher rate of coagulopathy, and the combination of vasoconstriction and hypovolemia at the time of TAE are thought to be the causes of this difference. There was no difference in mortality.

COMPLICATIONS OF TRANSCATHETER ARTERIAL EMBOLIZATION

Potential complications of TAE include contrast nephropathy, vascular injury at the puncture site or access vessel, nontarget embolization, and bowel ischemia. The overall reported adverse events rate is 6% to 9%,[77] and of major adverse events less than 2%.[40] Others have reported ischemic adverse events to be more common, occurring in 7% to 16% of cases.[78,79] Ischemic adverse events usually occur close to the time of TAE, or after a long delay (duodenal stenosis). Early bowel ischemia is commonly subclinical or of minimal sequalae. Late duodenal stenosis was more frequent in patients treated by NBCA, although it was proposed that the occlusion of terminal muscular branches rather than the particular agent was the cause.

A fatal case of acute necrotic pancreatitis localized to the pancreatic head region complicating TAE of the GDA and IPDA has also been reported.[80]

SUMMARY AND FUTURE HORIZONS

Teaching points related to this discussion are summarized in **Box 1**.

TAE is a viable option for cases of NVUGIB failing endoscopy, particularly in the setting of massive acute hemorrhage in poor operative candidates. Advances in catheter and wire technology, the development of a wide range of embolic materials, and modern interventional radiology angiography suites (with and without cone beam CT) has extended the ability of this technique, including patients with coagulopathy.

In the setup of a coagulopathic patient, interventional radiologists should be more frequently using NBCA and Onyx, given the rapidity to hemostasis. Embolization should be performed as close as possible to the bleeding point. Extent of superselective catheterization is limited by the size of available microcatheters. Koganemaru and colleagues[81] recently reported a trial in which a 1.7F microcatheter and 0.010-inch detachable coils were successfully deployed in small bowel vasa recta in 5 cases.

Box 1
TAE for nonvariceal upper GI bleeding: teaching points

1. The typical patient is hemodynamically unstable with massive bleeding resistant to medical management and endoscopic intervention.

2. Extravasation and/or mucosal blush are identified only in slightly more than one-half of cases. Extravasation is more likely to be identified in the presence of hemodynamic instability and significant transfusion requirements.

3. The risk of bowel ischemia as a complication of TAE in the upper GI tract is considerably less than that of the lower GI tract vasculature owing to the presence of arterial arcades and by embolization as close as possible to the bleeding site.

4. When used alone, Gelfoam is associated with a higher early rebleed rate and, therefore, other additional agents should be deployed.

5. In the presence of coagulopathy, coils alone may not achieve hemostasis; thus, an additional agent is commonly required.

6. Rebleeding after TAE is common; one-half of the cases respond to repeat TAE. Causes of rebleeding include coagulopathy, involvement of more than one vascular territory, and tumor-related bleeding.

7. NBCA and Onyx provide rapid hemostasis not affected by coagulopathy and, therefore, should probably be used more frequently.

Abbreviations: GI, gastrointestinal; NBCA, *N*-Butyl-2-cyanoacrylate; TAE, transcatheter arterial embolization.

Laursen and colleagues[82] performed a randomized controlled trial in which 109 patients successfully treated endoscopically for hemorrhage related to ulcer disease were randomized to undergo no further treatment or prophylactic TAE of the bleeding artery within 24 hours. There was an observed trend of less rebleeding in the TAE group. Further study is needed to verify this observation.

Additional advancements expected to become more widespread in the future include the use of radial access, CT angiography fusion road map and guidance, and endovascular robotics.[83]

REFERENCES

1. Margulis AR, Heinbecker P, Bernard HR. Operative mesenteric arteriography in the search for the site of bleeding in unexplained gastrointestinal hemorrhage. Surgery 1960;48:534.
2. Baum S, Nusbaum N, Clearfield HR, et al. Angiography in the diagnosis of gastrointestinal bleeding. Arch Int Med 1967;119:116.
3. Rosch J, Gray RK, Grollman JH, et al. Selective arterial drug infusion in the management of acute gastrointestinal bleeding. Gastroenterology 1970;59:341.
4. Rosch J, Dotter CT, Antonovic R. Selective vasoconstrictor infusion in the management of arteriocapillary gastrointestinal hemorrhage. AJR Am J Roentgenol 1972;116:279.
5. Rosch J, Dotter CT, Brown M. Selective arterial embolization. A new method for control of gastrointestinal bleeding. Radiology 1972;102:303.
6. Nusbaum M, Baum S. Radiographic demonstration of unknown sites of gastrointestinal bleeding. Surg Forum 1963;14:374.
7. Kruger K, Heindel W, Dolken W, et al. Angiographic detection of gastrointestinal bleeding: an experimental comparison of conventional screen-film angiography and digital subtraction angiography. Invest Radiol 1996;31:451–7.
8. Zink SI, Ohki SK, Stein B, et al. Noninvasive evaluation of active lower gastrointestinal bleeding: comparison between contrast enhanced MDCT and ^{99m}Tc RBC scintigraphy. AJR Am J Roentgenol 2008;191:1107.
9. Artigas JM, Martí M, Soto JA, et al. Multidetector CT angiography for acute gastrointestinal bleeding: technique and findings. Radiographics 2013;33(5):1453–70.
10. Kuhle WG, Sheiman RG. Detection of active colonic hemorrhage with use of helical CT: findings in a swine model. Radiology 2003;228:743.
11. Keller FS, Rosch J. Gastrointestinal hemorrhage. In: Geschwind JFH, Dake MD, editors. Abrams' angiography. Philadelphia: Wolters Kluwer/Lippincott Williams & Wilkins; 2014. p. 862–73.
12. Wu LM, Xu JR, Yin Y, et al. Usefulness of CT angiography in diagnosing acute gastrointestinal bleeding: a meta-analysis. World J Gastroenterol 2010;16:3957.
13. Heiss P, Zorger H, Hamer O, et al. Optimized multidetector computed tomography protocol for the diagnosis of active obscure gastrointestinal bleeding: a feasibility study. J Comput Assist Tomogr 2009;33:698.
14. Geffroy Y, Rodallec MH, Boulay-Coletta I, et al. Multidetector CT angiography in gastrointestinal bleeding: why, when and how. Radiographics 2011;31:831.
15. Yoon W, Jeong YY, Shin SS, et al. Acute massive gastrointestinal bleeding: detection and localization with arterial phase multi-detector row helical CT. Radiology 2006;239:160.
16. García-Blázquez V, Vicente-Bártulos A, Olavarria- Delgado A, et al. Accuracy of CT angiography in the diagnosis of acute gastrointestinal bleeding: systematic review and meta-analysis. Eur Radiol 2013;23:1181–90.

17. Kennedy DW, Laing CJ, Tseng LH, et al. Detection of active gastrointestinal hemorrhage with CT angiography: a 41/2-year retrospective review. J Vasc Interv Radiol 2010;21:848–55.

18. Singh-Bhinder N, Kim DH, Holly BP, et al. ACR appropriateness guidelines nonvariceal upper gastrointestinal bleeding. J Am Coll Radiol 2017;14:S177–8.

19. Mueller K, Datta S, Hwang G, et al. Digital subtraction imaging and cone-beam C-arm CT imaging. [Chapter 1]. In Kim DS, Orron DE, Patel N, et al, editors. Vascular imaging and intervention. New Delhi (India): Jaypee Bros, in press.

20. Loffroy R, Guiu B, D'Athis P, et al. Arterial embolotherapy for endoscopically unmanageable acute gastroduodenal hemorrhage: predictors of early rebleeding. Clin Gastroenterol Hepatol 2009;7:515–23.

21. Zurkiya O, Walker TG. Angiographic evaluation and management of nonvariceal gastrointestinal hemorrhage. AJR Am J Roentgenol 2015;205:753–63.

22. Loffroy R, Favelier S, Pottecher P, et al. Transcatheter arterial embolization for acute nonvariceal upper gastrointestinal bleeding: indications, techniques and outcomes. Diagn Interv Imaging 2015;96:731–44.

23. Kim CY, Guevara C, Orron DE, et al. Selective catheterization technique. [Chapter 24]. In Kim DS, Orron DE, Patel N, et al, editors. Vascular imaging and intervention. New Delhi (India): Jaypee Bros, in press.

24. Miyayama S, Matsui O, Akakura Y, et al. Use of a catheter with a large side hole for selective catheterization of the inferior phrenic artery. J Vasc Interv Radiol 2001;12(4):497–9.

25. Kiyosue H, Matsumoto S, Hori Y, et al. Turn-back technique with use of a shaped microcatheter for superselective catheterization of arteries originating at acute angles. J Vasc Interv Radiol 2004;15:641–3.

26. Baek JH, Chung JW, Jae HJ, et al. A new technique for superselective catheterization of arteries: preshaping of a micro-guide wire into a shepherd's hook form. Korean J Radiol 2007;8:225–30.

27. Morishita H, Takeuchi Y, Ito T, et al. Balloon Blocking Technique (BBT) for superselective catheterization of inaccessible arteries with conventional and modified techniques. Cardiovasc Intervent Radiol 2016;39(6):920–6.

28. Guevera CJ, Kim CY, Arya R, et al. Gastrointestinal hemorrhage. [Chapter 47]. In Kim DS, Orron DE, Patel N, et al, editors. Vascular imaging and intervention. New Delhi (India): Jaypee Bros, in press.

29. Kelemoridis V, Athanasoulis CA, Waltman CA. Gastric bleeding sites: an angiographic study. Radiology 1983;149:643.

30. Uflacker R. Atlas of vascular anatomy. An angiographic approach. 2nd edition. Philadelphia: Lippincott Williams & Wilkins; 2006.

31. Deso S, Howles GP, Orron DE, et al. Arterial anatomy of the abdomen and pelvis. [Chapter 12]. In. Kim DS, Orron DE, Patel N, et al, editors. Vascular imaging and intervention. New Delhi (India): Jaypee Bros, in press.

32. Miller M Jr, Smith TP. Angiographic diagnosis and endovascular management of nonvariceal gastrointestinal hemorrhage. Gastroenterol Clin North Am 2005;34:735–52.

33. Lee L, Iqbal S, Najmeh S, et al. Mesenteric angiography for acute gastrointestinal bleed: predictors of active extravasation and outcomes. Can J Surg 2012;55:382–8.

34. Aina R, Oliva VL, Therasse É, et al. Arterial embolotherapy for upper gastrointestinal hemorrhage: outcome assessment. J Vasc Interv Radiol 2001;12:195–200.

35. Schenker MP, Duszak R, Soulen MC, et al. Upper gastrointestinal hemorrhage and transcatheter embotherapy: clinical and technical factors impacting success and survival. J Vasc Interv Radiol 2001;12:1263.

36. Lang EV, Picus D, Marx MV, et al. Massive upper gastrointestinal hemorrhage with normal findings on arteriography; value of prophylactic embolization of the left gastric artery. AJR Am J Roentgenol 1992;158:547.
37. Padia SA, Geisinger MA, Newman JS, et al. Effectiveness of coil embolization in angiographically detectable versus non-detectable sources of upper gastrointestinal hemorrhage. J Vasc Interv Radiol 2009;20:461.
38. Pua U. Short- and long-term results of transcatheter embolization for massive arterial hemorrhage from gastroduodenal ulcers not controlled by endoscopic hemostasis. Can J Gastroenterol 2011;25(12):654.
39. Bloomfeld RS, Smith TP, Schneider AM, et al. Provocative angiography in patients with gastrointestinal hemorrhage of obscure origin. Am J Gastroenterol 2000;95: 2807–12.
40. Walker TG, Salazar GM, Waltman AC. Angiographic evaluation and management of acute gastrointestinal hemorrhage. World J Gastroenterol 2012;81:1191–201.
41. Ryan JM, Key SM, Dumbleton SA, et al. Nonlocalized lower gastrointestinal bleeding: provocative bleeding studies with intraarterial tPA, heparin, and tolazoline. J Vasc Interv Radiol 2001;12:1273–7.
42. Kim CY, Suhocki PV, Miller MJ Jr, et al. Provocative mesenteric angiography for lower gastrointestinal hemorrhage: results from a single-institution study. J Vasc Interv Radiol 2010;21(4):477–83.
43. Remzi FH, Dietz DW, Unal E, et al. Combined use of preoperative provocative angiography and highly selective methylene blue injection to localize an occult small-bowel bleeding site in a patient with Crohns disease. Report on a case. Dis Colon Rectum 2003;46:260.
44. Athanasoulis CA. The therapeutic applications of angiography. N Engl J Med 1980;302:1117.
45. Schmidt SP, Boskind JF, Smith DC, et al. Angiographic localization of small bowel angiodysplasia with use of platinum coils. J Vasc Interv Radiol 1993;4:737.
46. Dulai GS, Jensen DM, Kovacs TO, et al. Endoscopic treatment outcomes in watermelon stomach patients with and without portal hypertension. Endoscopy 2004;36:68–72.
47. Pryor AD, Pappas TN, Branch MS. Gastrointestinal bleeding: a practical approach to diagnosis and management. New York: Springer-Verlag; 2010.
48. Vrakas G, Pramateftakis MG, Raptis D, et al. Selective embolization for massive upper gastrointestinal bleeding delving from gastric angiodysplasia. JCSR 2012;3:11.
49. Khan R, Mahmad A, Gobrial M, et al. The diagnostic dilemma of Dieulafoy's lesion. Gastroenterology Res 2015;8:201–6.
50. Savides TJ, Jensen DM, Cohen J, et al. Severe upper gastrointestinal tumor bleeding: endoscopic findings, treatment, and outcome. Endoscopy 1996;28: 244–8.
51. Zandrino F, Tettoni SM, Gallesio I, et al. Emergency arterial embolization of upper gastrointestinal and jejunal tumors: an analysis of 12 patients with severe bleeding. Diagn Interv Imaging 2017;98:51–6.
52. Athanasoulis CA, Waltman AC, Novelline RA, et al. Angiography: its contribution to the emergency management of gastrointestinal hemorrhage. Radiol Clin North Am 1976;14:265.
53. Eckstein MR, Kelemouridis V, Athanasoulis CA, et al. Gastric bleeding: therapy with intraarterial vasopressin and transcatheter embolization. Radiology 1984; 152:643.
54. Kadir S, Athanasoulis CA. Angiographic management of gastrointestinal bleeding with vasopressin. Rofo 1977;127:111–9.

55. Keller FS, Rosch J. Angiography in the diagnosis and therapy of acute upper gastrointestinal bleeding. Schweiz Med Wochenschr 1979;109:586.

56. Porter DH, Kim D. Angiographic intervention in upper gastrointestinal bleeding. In: gastrointestinal emergencies. Baltimore (MD): Williams & Wilkins; 1997. p. 63–180.

57. Twiford TW, Granmayeh M, Tucker MJ. Gangrene of the feet associated with mesenteric intraarterial vasopressin. AJR Am J Roentgenol 1978;130:558.

58. Funaki B, Kostelic JK, Lorenz J, et al. Superselective microcoil embolization of colonic hemorrhage. AJR Am J Roentgenol 2001;177:829–36.

59. Walsworth M, Kim S, Gandhi RT, et al. Endovascular embolization devices, agents, and techniques. [Chapter 28]. In. Kim DS, Orron DE, Patel N, et al, editors. Vascular imaging and intervention. New Delhi (India): Jaypee Bros, in press.

60. Lang EV, Picus D, Marx VM, et al. Massive arterial hemorrhage from the stomach and lower esophagus: impact of embolotherapy on survival. Radiology 1990;177: 249–52.

61. Encarnacion CE, Kadir S, Beam CA, et al. Gastrointestinal bleeding: treatment with arterial embolization. Radiology 1992;183:505–8.

62. Rosch J, Keller FS, Kozak BE, et al. Gelfoam powder embolization of the left gastric artery in treatment of massive small vessel gastric bleeding. Radiology 1984;151:365.

63. Patel AA, Solomon JA, Soulen MC. Pharmaceuticals for intraarterial therapy. Semin Intervent Radiol 2005;22:130–8.

64. Lubarsky M, Ray CE, Funaki B. Embolization agents which one should be used when? Part 1: large vessel embolization. Semin Intervent Radiol 2009;26:352–7.

65. Toyoda H, Nakano S, Kumada T, et al. Estimation of usefulness of N-butyl-2-cyanoacrylate-lipiodol mixture in transcatheter arterial embolization for urgent control of life-threatening massive bleeding from gastric or duodenal ulcer. J Gastroenterol Hepatol 1996;11:252–8.

66. Lenhart M, Paetzel C, Sackmann M, et al. Superselective arterial embolisation with a liquid polyvinyl alcohol copolymer in patients with acute gastrointestinal haemorrhage. Eur Radiol 2010;20:1994–9.

67. Urbano J, Manuel Cabrera J, Franco A, et al. Selective arterial embolization with ethylene-vinyl alcohol copolymer for control of massive lower gastrointestinal bleeding: feasibility and initial experience. J Vasc Interv Radiol 2014;25:839–46.

68. Aoki M, Tokue H, Koyama Y, et al. Transcatheter arterial embolization with N-butyl cyanoacrylate for arterial esophageal bleeding in cancer patients. World J Surg Oncol 2016;14:54.

69. Patel TH, Cordts PR, Abcarian P, et al. Will transcatheter embolotherapy replace surgery in the treatment of gastrointestinal bleeding? Curr Surg 2001;58:323–7.

70. Kruz SH, Finkenzeller T, Schreyer A, et al. Transcatheter arterial embolisation in upper gastrointestinal bleeding in a sample of 29 patients in a gastrointestinal referral center in Germany. Z Gastroenterol 2015;53(09):1071–9.

71. Lee HH, Park JM, Chun HJ, et al. Transcatheter arterial embolization for endoscopically unmanageable non-variceal upper gastrointestinal bleeding. Scand J Gastroenterol 2015;50(7):809–15.

72. Koo HJ, Shin JH, Kim HJ, et al. Clinical outcome of transcatheter arterial embolization with N-Butyl-2-cyanoacrylate for control of acute gastrointestinal tract bleeding. AJR Am J Roentgenol 2015;204:662–8.

73. Heller SJ, Tokar JL, Nguyen MT, et al. Management of bleeding GI tumors. Gastrointest Endosc 2010;72:817–24.

74. Pereira J, Phan T. Management of bleeding in patients with advanced cancer. Oncologist 2004;9:561–70.
75. Yarris JP, Warden CR. Gastrointestinal bleeding in the cancer patient. Emerg Med Clin North Am 2009;27:363–79.
76. Beggs AD, Dilworth MP, Powell SL, et al. A systematic review of transarterial embolization versus emergency surgery in treatment of major nonvariceal upper gastrointestinal bleeding. Clin Exp Gastroenterol 2014;7:93–104.
77. Lundgren JA, Matsushima K, Lynch FC, et al. Angiographic embolization of non-variceal upper gastrointestinal bleeding: predictors of clinical failure. J Trauma 2011;70(5):1208–12.
78. Lang EK. Transcatheter embolization in management of hemorrhage from duodenal ulcer: long-term results and complications. Radiology 1992;182:703–7.
79. Poultsides GA, Kim CJ, Orlando R, et al. Angiographic embolization for gastroduodenal hemorrhage: safety, efficacy, and predictors of outcome. Arch Surg 2008; 143(5):457–61.
80. Matta A, Tandra PK, Cichowski E, et al. Acute necrotising pancreatitis: a late and fatal complication of pancreaticoduodenal arterial embolisation. BMJ Case Rep 2014;2014 [pi:bcr2014204197].
81. Koganemaru M, Nonoshita M, Iwamoto R, et al. Ultraselective embolization using a 1.7-Fr catheter and soft bare coil for small intestinal bleeding. Minim Invasive Ther Allied Technol 2016;25:345–50.
82. Laursen SB, Hansen JM, Andersen PE, et al. Supplementary arterial embolization an option in high-risk ulcer bleeding-a randomized study. Scand J Gastroenterol 2014;49:75–83.
83. Rao S, MacNamara F. Endovascular robotics. [Chapter 29]. In. Kim DS, Orron DE, Patel N, et al, editors. Vascular imaging and intervention. New Delhi (India): Jaypee Bros, in press.

Managing Antithrombotic Agents in the Setting of Acute Gastrointestinal Bleeding

Moe H. Kyaw, MBBS, MSc[a], Francis K.L. Chan, MD[b],*

KEYWORDS

- Antithrombotic agents • Gastrointestinal bleeding • Anticoagulants

KEY POINTS

- In general, if hemostasis is certain, antithrombotics should be resumed as soon as possible.
- This is because the outcome of a thrombotic event is usually far worse than a recurrent gastrointestinal (GI) bleeding event.
- Dilemmas arise when the clinician is not confident in whether hemostasis has been achieved.
- This is when the thrombotic risk assessment is required before a decision is made to withhold further antithrombotics.
- When the thrombotic risk is higher than the risk of recurrent GI bleeding, the antithrombotic agent should be continued.

INTRODUCTION

Antithrombotic-associated gastrointestinal (GI) bleeding is an increasing burden due to the growing population of advanced age, with multiple medical comorbidities, and the use of combinations of antiplatelet agents and anticoagulants.[1] GI bleeding in antithrombotic users is associated with subsequent increase in short-term and long-term mortality.[2] This increased mortality risk can be due to the disruption of antithrombotic or myocardial ischemia resulting from severe anemia or hemodynamic shock.

Although there may be consensus on ceasing anticoagulant and antiplatelet agents during an acute GI bleeding episode, debate remains concerning the appropriate approach to restarting these agents.[3–7] Clearer guidance is still needed on (1) under what circumstances each of the antiplatelet agents or anticoagulants should be stopped and (2) under what circumstances each of the antiplatelets or anticoagulants

[a] Department of Medicine & Therapeutics, Prince of Wales Hospital, The Chinese University of Hong Kong, 30-32 Ngan Shing Street, Shatin, Hong Kong; [b] Department of Medicine & Therapeutics, Prince of Wales Hospital, 30-32 Ngan Shing Street, Shatin, Hong Kong
* Corresponding author.
E-mail address: fklchan@cuhk.edu.hk

Gastrointest Endoscopy Clin N Am 28 (2018) 351–361
https://doi.org/10.1016/j.giec.2018.02.007
1052-5157/18/© 2018 Elsevier Inc. All rights reserved.

should be resumed, together with a time frame. This article provides the available evidence for the optimal management strategy of antithrombotics in the setting of acute GI bleeding and highlights areas weak in evidence in which future studies will be valuable.

GENERAL APPROACH TO THE MANAGEMENT OF ANTITHROMBOTICS

The following general approach can be adopted when faced with a patient with antithrombotic-associated bleeding:

1. Preendoscopy: (1) Resuscitation with fluids and blood, (2) assessing the need for reversing anticoagulant effects, and (3) early endoscopy.
2. Postendoscopy: An assessment should be made whether to continue or disrupt the antithrombotic based on a risk assessment: (1) What is the risk of recurrent bleeding after the endoscopic procedure? (2) What is the risk of a thrombotic event if the antithrombotic is disrupted?

MANAGEMENT OF ANTICOAGULANTS IN ACUTE GASTROINTESTINAL BLEEDING
Patients Receiving Warfarin

Summary

- Fresh frozen plasma (FFP) or prothrombin complex concentrate (PCC) should be the first-line reversal treatment of warfarin-associated bleeding.
- There are no randomized trials to assess whether or when warfarin should be resumed. The authors propose that in patients at high-risk for thrombosis (mechanical mitral valve, atrial fibrillation [AF] with CHADS$_2$ [congestive heart failure, hypertension, age $\geq$75 years, diabetes mellitus, stroke (double weight)] score 5 or 6, AF with rheumatic valvular heart disease, venous thromboembolism [VTE] within 3 months) warfarin should be resumed when definitive endoscopic hemostasis has been achieved. Concurrent heparin bridging therapy should be used until therapeutic INR have been achieved.
- When there is uncertainty concerning definitive endoscopic hemostasis, a second-look endoscopy can aid the decision on resumption of an antithrombotic agent.
- With the lack of high-quality evidence, it remains difficult to determine the time frame between thrombus formation and the subsequent clinical event and cessation of anticoagulant. Further research is required to identify the optimal duration of warfarin interruption after a GI bleeding episode.

Reversing the anticoagulant effects of warfarin
The most commonly used anticoagulant remains warfarin. The half-life of warfarin is approximately 40 hours. If the INR is between 2.0 and 3.0, it will require 4 days for the INR to reduce to 1.5 after withdrawal.[8]

Warfarin anticoagulant effect can be reversed with intravenous (IV) vitamin K or FFP or PCC. Vitamin K promotes the synthesis of new clotting factors II, VII, IX, and X. The INR will decrease within 2 to 4 hours following IV vitamin K infusion and normalize within 24 hours. FFP is a blood product made from the liquid portion of whole blood. The recommended adult therapeutic dose is 12 to 15 mL/kg. The effect of FFP will start in 10 minutes but it may take a few hours to show reversal of INR and up to 9 hours before the complete reversal of INR.[9]

Prothrombin complex concentrate PCC is a pharmacologic product made up of clotting factors II, IX, and X. Different processing techniques enable the production of either 3-factor (factors II, IX, and X) or 4-factor (factors II, VII, IX, and X) concentrates. The advantages of PCC compared with FFP include reduced volume, room-temperature storage, and lack of requirement of blood type matching. The major drawback of PCC has been the risk of thrombotic complications. Current evidence from a meta-analysis suggests the incidence of thrombotic events to be 0.7% and 1.8% in patients treated with 3-factor PCC and 4-factor PCC, respectively.[10]

Other anticoagulant reversal blood products Recombinant factor VIIa (rFVIIa) is a pharmacologic product similar to native factor VIIa. It causes activation of the extrinsic pathway of blood coagulation. It is cleared by the US Food and Drug Administration (FDA) for treatment of bleeding episodes in hemophilia. With its associated high thrombotic risk,[11] its routine use should be avoided until better quality evidence is available.

Whether FFP or PCC should be the first-line reversal treatment of warfarin-associated bleeding is not yet determined. In a Cochrane meta-analysis there was no statistical significance in mortality between the uses of PCC and FFP in warfarin-associated bleeding.[12]

What is the optimal international normalized ratio before endoscopy? What the optimal INR should be before endoscopy is performed remains unknown. Endoscopic hemostasis has been successfully achieved in patients with an INR between 1.5 and 2.5.[13] It is not necessary to completely normalize the INR before endoscopy because this does not reduce the bleeding risk and only delays endoscopy.

Thrombotic risk after disruption of warfarin: when to resume warfarin
The risk of thromboembolism if warfarin is disrupted depends on the indication for warfarin therapy and the individual risk of patient.[14] A meta-analysis concluded that resumption of warfarin following disruption after GI bleeding was associated with a reduction in thrombotic events (hazard ratio [HR] 0.68, 95% CI 0.52–0.88) and mortality (HR 0.76, 95% CI 0.66–0.88) without a statistically significant increase in recurrent GI bleeding (HR 1.20, 95% CI 0.97–1.48).[15]

There are few data concerning the optimal timing of warfarin resumption. Of the studies that compared adverse events in patients who resumed warfarin and those who remained off anticoagulation after bleeding,[16–18] only Qureshi and colleagues[16] assessed the time frame for adverse events. For recurrent GI bleeding, the group for whom warfarin was resumed within 7 days had a 2-fold increased risk of bleeding; however, there was no significant difference in the risk of bleeding between resuming warfarin after 7 days of interruption of warfarin compared with resuming warfarin after 30 days.

Should heparin bridging be initiated if warfarin is disrupted?
When warfarin is disrupted, bridging anticoagulation can be provided by administration of a short-acting anticoagulant of either low-molecular-weight heparin or unfractionated heparin. Unfractionated heparin administered intravenously has a half-life of 60 to 90 minutes and its anticoagulant effect disappears after 3 to 4 hours.

The benefit of heparin bridging in patients with AF remains unproven. The role of heparin bridging has mostly been assessed in the elective perioperative setting. A meta-analysis reported no difference in thrombotic risk between bridged and non-bridged groups (odds ratio [OR] 0.80, 95% CI 0.42–1.54) but heparin bridging significantly increased the risk of bleeding (OR 5.40, 95% CI 3.00–9.74).[19]

The authors propose that in patients at highest risk of thrombosis (mechanical mitral valve, AF with CHADS$_2$ score 5 or 6, AF with rheumatic valvular heart disease, VTE within 3 months) warfarin should be resumed when endoscopic hemostasis has been achieved, together with heparin bridging therapy until a therapeutic INR is reached.

Patients Receiving Direct-Acting Oral Anticoagulants

Summary

- If the last dose of direct-acting oral anticoagulants (DOACs) was taken more than 12 hours before and patient does not have predisposing factors for excessive levels of DOACs, a reversal agent is unlikely to be beneficial.
- PCC is the only blood product that may be effective in reversing the anticoagulant effect of DOAC; there is no evidence for FFP or IV vitamin K.
- Idarucizumab (for dabigatran) is the only available antidote.
- Heparin bridging is not required following DOAC-associated GI bleeding.
- When resuming DOACs, clinicians should be aware that their full anticoagulant effect could occur within 4 hours.

The 2 types of DOAC currently available are inhibitors of thrombin (dabigatran) and inhibitors of coagulation factor Xa (rivaroxaban, apixaban, edoxaban). They are indicated for patients with AF or VTE but not for patients with mechanical heart valves.

Major differences between the management of gastrointestinal bleeding associated with warfarin and direct-acting oral anticoagulants

1. If there is no renal or liver impairment the disappearance of the anticoagulant effect of DOACs after their stoppage is predictable (duration 12 to 24 hours) and a reversal agent may not be required.
2. Routine laboratory tests do not reliably measure the anticoagulant effects of DOACs.

Unlike warfarin, which blocks the formation of vitamin K–dependent coagulation factors, DOAC blocks a single step in the coagulation cascade. Monitoring the anticoagulation effects of DOACS is challenging because activated partial thromboplastin time and prothrombin time do not provide accurate measures of coagulation. For dabigatran, the degree of coagulation can be assessed by the ecarin clotting time or dilute thrombin time. For other DOACs, drug-specific anti-Xa factor assays can be used. However, these tests are not commonly available.

Gastrointestinal bleeding risk with direct-acting oral anticoagulants

Although DOACS have a lower overall risk of major bleeding, both dabigatran[20] and rivaroxaban[21] have higher incidences of GI bleeding compared with warfarin. Apixaban is thought to have the lowest GI bleeding risk. A meta-analysis involving 4 randomized trials with a total of 42,411 subjects suggested that DOACs have significantly reduced all-cause mortality (relative risk [RR] 0.90, 95% CI 0.85–0.95) and intracranial hemorrhage (RR 0.48, 95% CI 0.39–0.59) but increased GI bleeding (RR 1.25, 95% CI 1.01–1.55).[22] When examining the risk of individual DOACs, apixaban had the lowest GI bleeding risk among the DOACs and the risk was lower than warfarin (HR 0.89, CI 95% 0.70–1.15).

Who are at risk of excessive blood levels of direct-acting oral anticoagulants?

The blood levels of DOACs can be affected by last dosing of DOAC, creatinine clearance, body weight, and gender (female). In a DOAC user presenting with GI bleeding, if the last dose was taken more than 12 hours earlier, and the patient does not have predisposing factors for excessive levels of DOAC, it is unlikely that the bleeding episode is attributed to DOAC. Therefore, using a reversal agent may not be beneficial in this setting.

It may be valuable to measure DOAC levels in patients with risk factors for excessive blood levels of DOACs, including

1. Extreme body weight: The pharmacokinetics and pharmacodynamics of DOACs (more so with factor Xa inhibitors) may be affected by extreme body weights (<50 kg, >120 kg, or body mass index $\geq$35 kg/m^2).[23]
2. Concomitant drugs: Each DOAC is a substrate of permeability-glycoprotein (P-gp).[24] Hepatic enzyme cytochrome P450 3A4 (CYP3A4) metabolizes rivaroxaban, apixaban, and edoxaban (not dabigatran). There is a long list of P-gp inhibitors. Of commonly used drugs, this includes antiarrhythmic drugs (amiodarone, verapamil, diltiazem) and antimicrobials (clarithromycin, erythromycin, ketoconazole). Commonly used drugs that both inhibit P-gp and CYP3A4 include clarithromycin, ketoconazole, cyclosporine, and tamoxifen.[25]
3. Renal impairment (creatinine clearance <50 mL/min): All DOACs have various degrees of renal excretion. Patients with renal impairment are at higher risk of DOAC-associated bleeding.[26]
4. Advanced liver disease: The anticoagulant effect is increased with increasing severity of liver disease.[27] Clinical evidence remains limited because many of the initial clinical trials on DOACs excluded patients with advanced liver disease.

Reversing the anticoagulant effects of direct-acting oral anticoagulants
The following reversal strategies can be considered if a patient is presumed to be at risk for excessive levels of DOACs, although evidence remains limited:

1. Gastric lavage and oral charcoal: Consider if DOAC was taken within 2 to 3 hours before. Evidence is only available for dabigatran[28] and none exists for factor Xa inhibitors.
2. Blood products: PCC may be considered but evidence is available only from healthy volunteers without bleeding.[29,30] There is no evidence for the use of vitamin K or FFP for reversing the effects of DOACs. The effect of PCC[31] and rFVIIa[32] for reversal of the anticoagulant effects of DOACs has only been shown in healthy volunteers without bleeding. With rFVIIa presumed to have a higher risk of thrombosis, it should be considered only as a second-line reversal treatment after failure of PCC or activated PCC.
3. Hemodialysis: Hemodialysis may reverse the anticoagulant effect of dabigatran due to the low protein-binding nature of this drug (35%).[33] Hemodialysis is not effective with other DOACs such as rivaroxaban and apixaban because these drugs are highly protein bound, 95% and 87%, respectively.[34]
4. Antidotes: Idarucizumab for dabigatran is the only antidote currently available and cleared for use by the FDA.[35] There are several DOAC-antidotes undergoing development (eg, andexanet alfa, ciraparantag).

Thrombotic risk after disruption of direct-acting oral anticoagulants: when to resume direct-acting oral anticoagulants
Sherwood and colleagues[36] conducted a subgroup analysis of the ROCKET AF study [Rivaroxaban Once Daily Oral Direct Factor Xa Inhibition Compared with Vitamin K Antagonism for Prevention of Stroke and Embolism Trial in Atrial Fibrillation] to determine the outcomes of subjects in whom anticoagulant use (rivaroxaban or warfarin) was interrupted (3–30 days) for any reason. The rate for thrombotic events during the anticoagulant-interrupted period was similar in the rivaroxaban and warfarin groups (0.30% vs 0.41% per 30 days, HR 0.74, 95% CI 0.36–1.50).

A prospective, open-label study assessed idarucizumab for reversing the anticoagulant effect of dabigatran for patients who had uncontrolled bleeding or were about to undergo an urgent procedure. Twenty-four of the 403 subjects (4.8%) developed a thrombotic event within 30 days after reversal treatment and 34 subjects (6.8%) within 90 days after treatment.[37] All the thrombotic events that occurred within 3 days after reversal of anticoagulation occurred in subjects in whom anticoagulation had not been restarted.

Should heparin bridging be initiated if direct-acting oral anticoagulants therapy was disrupted?

In a prospective observational study of patients receiving DOAC and undergoing interventional procedures, heparin bridging did not reduce cardiovascular events but led to significantly higher rates of major bleeding complications (2.7%, 95% CI 1.1–5.5) compared with no bridging (0.5%, 95% 0.1–1.4, $P = .010$).[38] Subgroup analysis of a randomized trial comparing dabigatran versus warfarin in patients with AF[20] reported an increased incidence of bleeding with heparin bridging, without a reduction in thromboembolism (6.8% vs 1.8%).[39,40] Current evidence does not support the use of heparin bridging in patients on DOACs.

MANAGEMENT OF ANTIPLATELETS IN ACUTE GASTROINTESTINAL BLEEDING
Patients Receiving Aspirin Monotherapy

Summary

- Aspirin should be continued in patients receiving aspirin monotherapy following acute GI bleeding if endoscopic hemostasis has been achieved.

Thrombotic risk after disruption of aspirin monotherapy: should aspirin be disrupted?

Both aspirin and clopidogrel prevent thrombus formation by irreversibly inhibiting platelet function. After each day of interruption of antiplatelet agent, 10-14% of the platelet function is restored each day, and it takes 7 days for the whole platelet pool to be replaced.[40] The risk of a thrombotic event without aspirin therapy is 10-fold higher in secondary Cardiovascular (CV) prevention than in primary CV prevention (3.11% vs 0.34%, yearly).[41] In a meta-analysis of observational studies (6 studies) predominantly focusing on adherence to aspirin therapy in secondary CV prevention, aspirin cessation was associated with a 2-fold risk of a thrombotic event (OR 3.14, 95% CI 1.75–5.61). In the only randomized study addressing the management of aspirin after GI bleeding (subjects receiving aspirin for secondary CV prevention and presenting with acute upper GI bleeding), the rate of CV events was higher in those who stopped aspirin.[42] The authors propose that aspirin should be continued if endoscopic hemostasis has been achieved.

Patients Receiving Dual Antiplatelet Therapy with Aspirin and Clopidogrel

Summary

- In patients with dual antiplatelet therapy (DAPT), clopidogrel may be disrupted for 5 to 7 days as long as aspirin is continued.

Thrombotic risk after disruption of dual antiplatelet therapy: should aspirin and/or clopidogrel be disrupted?

The highest risk thrombotic events are within the following circumstances; therefore, altering DAPT during these periods is best avoided[43–45]:

1. Within the first 6 months after an acute coronary syndrome
2. Within first 30 to 45 days after insertion of bare metal stents
3. Within first 6 months after insertion of drug-eluting stents.

In a large prospective observational study of 5031 subjects who had coronary stenting, subjects were followed up to assess the risk of cessation of DAPT. The thrombotic risk was highest within the 7 days after cessation (HR 7.04, 95% CI 3.31–14.95).[46] In a subgroup analysis, the thrombotic risk was numerically higher when discontinuation or disruption occurred with both medications versus only 1 antiplatelet medication.

In a meta-analysis assessing the risk of short-term discontinuation of DAPT in subjects with drug-eluting stents, when subjects stopped both antiplatelet agents simultaneously, the median time to an event was 7 days, whereas if clopidogrel was stopped but aspirin was maintained, the median time to an event was 122 days. This study concluded that if aspirin therapy is maintained, short-term discontinuation of clopidogrel might be relatively safe in patients with drug-eluting stents.[44]

Decision on resumption of antiplatelet agents also depends on the type of coronary stent. Second-generation drug-eluting stents (everolimus-eluting, zotarolimus-eluting) have a lower risk of stent thrombosis compared with first-generation drug-eluting stents. Randomized studies have suggested that short DAPT durations of 3 to 6 months could be safe with second-generation drug-eluting stents.[47,48] Thus, if bleeding occurs after 3 to 6 months after placement of these second-generation stents, clopidogrel may be discontinued while continuing aspirin. Furthermore, with the newest stents, such as the polymer-free umirolimus-coated stents, 30 days of DAPT may even be adequate to prevent thrombosis.[49]

Patients Receiving Newer Antiplatelet Agents (Ticagrelor, Prasugrel, Vorapaxar)

Despite weak evidence, the newer antiplatelet agents are perceived to have a higher risk of bleeding than clopidogrel. The highest bleeding risk is suggested to be with vorapaxar.[50] There are no data on the disruption and resumption of the ADP receptor inhibitors, such as prasugrel, ticagrelor, or protease-activated receptor-1 inhibitor vorapaxar.

Patients Receiving Triple Therapy (2 Antiplatelet Agents and an Anticoagulant)

There will be patients who had acute coronary syndrome with or without stenting and have AF, who will require DAPT for a period of 1 year and long-term warfarin. These patients are at considerable risk of GI bleeding and present a great challenge to clinicians.[51] The crude incidence of major bleeding ranges from 3% to 16% from clinical studies.[51,52] Using clopidogrel without aspirin was associated with a significant reduction in bleeding complications (HR 0.36, 95% CI 0.26–0.50, $P<.0001$) and no increase in the rate of thrombotic events.[53] Based on these studies, it may be reasonable for disruption of 1 of the antiplatelet agents (not clopidogrel after first month of stent insertion) while continuing the anticoagulant.

SUMMARY

In general, if hemostasis is certain, antithrombotics should be resumed as soon as possible. This is because the outcome of a thrombotic event is usually far worse than a recurrent GI bleeding event. Dilemmas arise when the clinician is not confident in whether hemostasis has been achieved. This is when the thrombotic risk assessment is required before a decision is made to withhold further antithrombotics. When the thrombotic risk is higher than the risk of recurrent GI bleeding, the antithrombotic agent should be continued. When the bleeding risk is higher than the thrombotic risk, cessation of the antithrombotic agent may be appropriate.

Although there are several scores to predict the risk of recurrent GI bleeding after upper GI bleeding, whether these can inform which patients can safely continue antithrombotics remains to be proven. Like many other recommendations on management of antithrombotics in acute GI bleeding, these are based on expert opinion. Despite the numerous occasions of patients presenting to hospitals with antithrombotic-associated bleeding, there remains a lack of prospective trials.

REFERENCES

1. Go AS, Mozaffarian D, Roger VL, et al. Heart disease and stroke statistics–2013 update: a report from the American Heart Association. Circulation 2013;127(1): e6–245.
2. Lopes RD, Subherwal S, Holmes DN, et al. The association of in-hospital major bleeding with short-, intermediate-, and long-term mortality among older patients with non-ST-segment elevation myocardial infarction. Eur Heart J 2012;33(16): 2044–53.
3. Laine L, Jensen DM. Management of patients with ulcer bleeding. Am J Gastroenterol 2012;107(3):345–60 [quiz: 361].
4. Barkun AN, Bardou M, Kuipers EJ, et al. International consensus recommendations on the management of patients with nonvariceal upper gastrointestinal bleeding. Ann Intern Med 2010;152(2):101–13.
5. Laursen SB, Jorgensen HS, Schaffalitzky de Muckadell OB, Danish Society of Gastroenterology and Hepatology. Management of bleeding gastroduodenal ulcers. Dan Med J 2012;59(7):C4473.
6. Veitch AM, Baglin TP, Gershlick AH, et al. Guidelines for the management of anticoagulant and antiplatelet therapy in patients undergoing endoscopic procedures. Gut 2008;57(9):1322–9.
7. Gralnek IM, Dumonceau JM, Kuipers EJ, et al. Diagnosis and management of nonvariceal upper gastrointestinal hemorrhage: European Society of Gastrointestinal Endoscopy (ESGE) Guideline. Endoscopy 2015;47(10):a1–46.
8. White RH, McKittrick T, Hutchinson R, et al. Temporary discontinuation of warfarin therapy: changes in the international normalized ratio. Ann Intern Med 1995; 122(1):40–2.
9. Holland LL, Brooks JP. Toward rational fresh frozen plasma transfusion: the effect of plasma transfusion on coagulation test results. Am J Clin Pathol 2006;126(1): 133–9.
10. Dentali F, Marchesi C, Giorgi Pierfranceschi M, et al. Safety of prothrombin complex concentrates for rapid anticoagulation reversal of vitamin K antagonists. A meta-analysis. Thromb Haemost 2011;106(3):429–38.
11. O'Connell KA, Wood JJ, Wise RP, et al. Thromboembolic adverse events after use of recombinant human coagulation factor VIIa. JAMA 2006;295(3):293–8.
12. Johansen M, Wikkelso A, Lunde J, et al. Prothrombin complex concentrate for reversal of vitamin K antagonist treatment in bleeding and non-bleeding patients. Cochrane Database Syst Rev 2015;(7):CD010555.
13. Choudari CP, Rajgopal C, Palmer KR. Acute gastrointestinal haemorrhage in anticoagulated patients: diagnoses and response to endoscopic treatment. Gut 1994;35(4):464–6.
14. Douketis JD, Spyropoulos AC, Spencer FA, et al. Perioperative management of antithrombotic therapy: antithrombotic therapy and prevention of thrombosis, 9th ed: American College of Chest Physicians Evidence-Based Clinical Practice Guidelines. Chest 2012;141(2 Suppl):e326S–50S.
15. Chai-Adisaksopha C, Hillis C, Monreal M, et al. Thromboembolic events, recurrent bleeding and mortality after resuming anticoagulant following gastrointestinal bleeding. A meta-analysis. Thromb Haemost 2015;114(4):819–25.

16. Qureshi W, Mittal C, Patsias I, et al. Restarting anticoagulation and outcomes after major gastrointestinal bleeding in atrial fibrillation. Am J Cardiol 2014;113(4): 662–8.
17. Nieto JA, Camara T, Gonzalez-Higueras E, et al. Clinical outcome of patients with major bleeding after venous thromboembolism. Findings from the RIETE registry. Thromb Haemost 2008;100(5):789–96.
18. Witt DM, Delate T, Garcia DA, et al. Risk of thromboembolism, recurrent hemorrhage, and death after warfarin therapy interruption for gastrointestinal tract bleeding. Arch Intern Med 2012;172(19):1484–91.
19. Siegal D, Yudin J, Kaatz S, et al. Periprocedural heparin bridging in patients receiving vitamin K antagonists: systematic review and meta-analysis of bleeding and thromboembolic rates. Circulation 2012;126(13):1630–9.
20. Connolly SJ, Ezekowitz MD, Yusuf S, et al. Dabigatran versus warfarin in patients with atrial fibrillation. N Engl J Med 2009;361(12):1139–51.
21. Patel MR, Mahaffey KW, Garg J, et al. Rivaroxaban versus warfarin in nonvalvular atrial fibrillation. N Engl J Med 2011;365(10):883–91.
22. Ruff CT, Giugliano RP, Braunwald E, et al. Comparison of the efficacy and safety of new oral anticoagulants with warfarin in patients with atrial fibrillation: a meta-analysis of randomised trials. Lancet 2014;383(9921):955–62.
23. Upreti VV, Wang J, Barrett YC, et al. Effect of extremes of body weight on the pharmacokinetics, pharmacodynamics, safety and tolerability of apixaban in healthy subjects. Br J Clin Pharmacol 2013;76(6):908–16.
24. Wessler JD, Grip LT, Mendell J, et al. The P-glycoprotein transport system and cardiovascular drugs. J Am Coll Cardiol 2013;61(25):2495–502.
25. Gong IY, Kim RB. Importance of pharmacokinetic profile and variability as determinants of dose and response to dabigatran, rivaroxaban, and apixaban. Can J Cardiol 2013;29(7 Suppl):S24–33.
26. Fountzilas C, George J, Levine R. Dabigatran overdose secondary to acute kidney injury and amiodarone use. N Z Med J 2013;126(1370):110–2.
27. Kubitza D, Roth A, Becka M, et al. Effect of hepatic impairment on the pharmacokinetics and pharmacodynamics of a single dose of rivaroxaban, an oral, direct Factor Xa inhibitor. Br J Clin Pharmacol 2013;76(1):89–98.
28. van Ryn J, Sieger P, Kink-Eiband M, et al. Adsorption of dabigatran etexilate in water or dabigatran in pooled human plasma by activated charcoal in vitro. Blood 2009;114(22): Abstract 1065.
29. Eerenberg ES, Kamphuisen PW, Sijpkens MK, et al. Reversal of rivaroxaban and dabigatran by prothrombin complex concentrate: a randomized, placebo-controlled, crossover study in healthy subjects. Circulation 2011;124(14):1573–9.
30. Escolar G, Fernandez-Gallego V, Arellano-Rodrigo E, et al. Reversal of apixaban induced alterations in hemostasis by different coagulation factor concentrates: significance of studies in vitro with circulating human blood. PLoS One 2013; 8(11):e78696.
31. Marlu R, Hodaj E, Paris A, et al. Effect of non-specific reversal agents on anticoagulant activity of dabigatran and rivaroxaban: a randomised crossover ex vivo study in healthy volunteers. Thromb Haemost 2012;108(2):217–24.
32. Khoo TL, Weatherburn C, Kershaw G, et al. The use of FEIBA(R) in the correction of coagulation abnormalities induced by dabigatran. Int J Lab Hematol 2013; 35(2):222–4.
33. Stangier J, Rathgen K, Stahle H, et al. Influence of renal impairment on the pharmacokinetics and pharmacodynamics of oral dabigatran etexilate: an open-label, parallel-group, single-centre study. Clin Pharmacokinet 2010;49(4):259–68.

34. Ieko M, Naitoh S, Yoshida M, et al. Profiles of direct oral anticoagulants and clinical usage-dosage and dose regimen differences. J Intensive Care 2016;4:19 [eCollection: 2016].

35. Pollack CV Jr, Reilly PA, Bernstein R, et al. Design and rationale for RE-VERSE AD: A phase 3 study of idarucizumab, a specific reversal agent for dabigatran. Thromb Haemost 2015;114(1):198–205.

36. Sherwood MW, Douketis JD, Patel MR, et al. Outcomes of temporary interruption of rivaroxaban compared with warfarin in patients with nonvalvular atrial fibrillation: results from the rivaroxaban once daily, oral, direct factor Xa inhibition compared with vitamin K antagonism for prevention of stroke and embolism trial in atrial fibrillation (ROCKET AF). Circulation 2014;129(18):1850–9.

37. Pollack CV Jr, Reilly PA, van Ryn J, et al. Idarucizumab for dabigatran reversal - full cohort analysis. N Engl J Med 2017;377(5):431–41.

38. Beyer-Westendorf J, Gelbricht V, Forster K, et al. Peri-interventional management of novel oral anticoagulants in daily care: results from the prospective Dresden NOAC registry. Eur Heart J 2014;35(28):1888–96.

39. Douketis JD, Healey JS, Brueckmann M, et al. Perioperative bridging anticoagulation during dabigatran or warfarin interruption among patients who had an elective surgery or procedure. Substudy of the RE-LY trial. Thromb Haemost 2015; 113(3):625–32.

40. Roth GJ, Majerus PW. The mechanism of the effect of aspirin on human platelets. I. Acetylation of a particulate fraction protein. J Clin Invest 1975;56(3):624–32.

41. Antithrombotic Trialists' (ATT) Collaboration, Baigent C, Blackwell L, Collins R, et al. Aspirin in the primary and secondary prevention of vascular disease: collaborative meta-analysis of individual participant data from randomised trials. Lancet 2009;373(9678):1849–60.

42. Sung JJ, Lau JY, Ching JY, et al. Continuation of low-dose aspirin therapy in peptic ulcer bleeding: a randomized trial. Ann Intern Med 2010;152(1):1–9.

43. van Werkum JW, Heestermans AA, Zomer AC, et al. Predictors of coronary stent thrombosis: the Dutch stent thrombosis registry. J Am Coll Cardiol 2009;53(16): 1399–409.

44. Eisenberg MJ, Richard PR, Libersan D, et al. Safety of short-term discontinuation of antiplatelet therapy in patients with drug-eluting stents. Circulation 2009; 119(12):1634–42.

45. Park DW, Park SW, Park KH, et al. Frequency of and risk factors for stent thrombosis after drug-eluting stent implantation during long-term follow-up. Am J Cardiol 2006;98(3):352–6.

46. Mehran R, Baber U, Steg PG, et al. Cessation of dual antiplatelet treatment and cardiac events after percutaneous coronary intervention (PARIS): 2 year results from a prospective observational study. Lancet 2013;382(9906):1714–22.

47. Kim BK, Hong MK, Shin DH, et al. A new strategy for discontinuation of dual antiplatelet therapy: the RESET Trial (REal Safety and Efficacy of 3-month dual antiplatelet Therapy following Endeavor zotarolimus-eluting stent implantation). J Am Coll Cardiol 2012;60(15):1340–8.

48. Valgimigli M, Campo G, Monti M, et al. Short- versus long-term duration of dual-antiplatelet therapy after coronary stenting: a randomized multicenter trial. Circulation 2012;125(16):2015–26.

49. Urban P, Meredith IT, Abizaid A, et al. Polymer-free drug-coated coronary stents in patients at high bleeding risk. N Engl J Med 2015;373(21):2038–47.

50. Morrow DA, Braunwald E, Bonaca MP, et al. Vorapaxar in the secondary prevention of atherothrombotic events. N Engl J Med 2012;366(15):1404–13.

51. Lamberts M, Olesen JB, Ruwald MH, et al. Bleeding after initiation of multiple an-
    tithrombotic drugs, including triple therapy, in atrial fibrillation patients following
    myocardial infarction and coronary intervention: a nationwide cohort study. Circu-
    lation 2012;126(10):1185–93.
52. Sorensen R, Hansen ML, Abildstrom SZ, et al. Risk of bleeding in patients with
    acute myocardial infarction treated with different combinations of aspirin, clopi-
    dogrel, and vitamin K antagonists in Denmark: a retrospective analysis of nation-
    wide registry data. Lancet 2009;374(9706):1967–74.
53. Dewilde WJ, Oirbans T, Verheugt FW, et al. Use of clopidogrel with or without
    aspirin in patients taking oral anticoagulant therapy and undergoing percuta-
    neous coronary intervention: an open-label, randomised, controlled trial. Lancet
    2013;381(9872):1107–15.

Patient Presentation, Risk Stratification, and Initial Management in Acute Lower Gastrointestinal Bleeding

Majid A. Almadi, MBBS, FRCPC, MSc (Clinical Epidemiology)[a,b],
Alan N. Barkun, MD, CM, FRCPC, MSc (Clinical Epidemiology)[b,c],*

KEYWORDS

- Gastrointestinal bleeding • Lower gastrointestinal bleeding • Diverticulosis
- Endoscopy • Colonoscopy

KEY POINTS

- The incidence of hospitalization for lower gastrointestinal bleeding has decreased marginally in the United States but remains a significant cause of morbidity and mortality.
- Causes of lower gastrointestinal bleeding vary depending on the age of patients as well as coexisting comorbid conditions.
- Risk stratification facilitates appropriate patient disposition as well as initiation of involvement of supportive teams and resource mobilization to, it is hoped, reduce morbidity and mortality.
- Initial resuscitation, including hemodynamic stabilization, is critical; laboratory investigations should also be undertaken during the initial patient assessment and patients' condition optimized before endoscopic intervention.
- The management of comorbid conditions, including the appropriate use of antiplatelet agents and anticoagulants, requires a multidisciplinary approach with individualized tailoring.

INTRODUCTION

About 30% to 40% of all cases of gastrointestinal bleeding originate from a lower gastrointestinal source[1]; although lower gastrointestinal bleeding (LGIB) used to be less common compared with upper gastrointestinal bleeding, this ratio has changed

[a] Division of Gastroenterology, King Khalid University Hospital, King Saud University, Riyadh, Saudi Arabia; [b] Division of Gastroenterology, The McGill University Health Center, Montreal General Hospital, McGill University, 1650 Cedar Avenue, Montreal, Quebec H3G 1A4, Canada; [c] Division of Clinical Epidemiology, The McGill University Health Center, Montreal General Hospital, McGill University, 1650 Cedar Avenue, Montreal, Quebec H3G 1A4, Canada
* Corresponding author. Montreal General Hospital, 1650 Cedar Avenue, #D7-148, Montreal, Quebec H3G 1A4, Canada.
E-mail address: alan.barkun@muhc.mcgill.ca

Gastrointest Endoscopy Clin N Am 28 (2018) 363–377
https://doi.org/10.1016/j.giec.2018.02.008

over time. Indeed, emergency department visits between 2007 and 2012 for upper gastrointestinal bleeding decreased by 5%, whereas those for LGIB increased by 17%, with about 900,000 ambulatory care visits in the United States in 2010.[1]

LGIB historically referred to any bleeding distal to the ligament of Treitz, but since 2006 this definition has been modified to bleeding from a source distal to the ileocecal valve.[2-4] The reader must, however, keep in mind that this change in nomenclature is recent and is not reflected in older literature.[5,6]

The management of LGIB has evolved over the last few years to incorporate a multi-disciplinary management strategy in which diagnostic tools like computed tomographic angiography as well as transarterial embolization play a larger role in caring for patients with LGIB.

This article provides a synopsis on the presentation of overt LGIB and the risk stratification of affected patients as well as reviews acute management issues based on the best evidence available to date.

EPIDEMIOLOGY

The age- and sex-adjusted incidence of hospitalization for LGIB has decreased marginally in the United States from 2001 to 2009 (41.8–35.7 per 100,000)[7] but remains a significant source of morbidity and mortality (case fatality rate of 1.47%). When compared with upper gastrointestinal bleeding, LGIB is associated with a higher mortality (8.8% vs 5.5%), longer hospital stay (11.6 ± 13.9 vs 7.9 ± 8.8 days), and greater resource utilization.[8] In England, 2.7% of all red blood cell transfusions countrywide are used for cases of LGIB.[9]

A national audit in the United Kingdom that incorporated 143 hospitals with a total of 2528 patients with LGIB who presented within 2 months in 2015 reported a median age presentation of 74 years, whereas most patients (79.1%) had coexisting comorbidities; a significant proportion of patients were receiving either oral anticoagulant (15.9%) or antiplatelet therapy (29.4%).[10]

In a recent systematic review and meta-analysis,[11] the overall mortality associated with LGIB was 0.4%, whereas the bleeding-related mortality was 1.1%. Furthermore, LGIB was associated with a recurrent bleeding rate of 13.5% (95% confidence interval [CI]; 11.8% to 15.5%); length of hospital and intensive care unit (ICU) stays were 5.7 ± 5.2 and 1.9 ± 0.4 days, respectively. Overall, 13.6% patients experienced further bleeding during their hospitalization, whereas 4.4% were readmitted with recurrent bleeding within 28 days.[10] The average total number of blood transfusions received by patients was 3.4 ± 2.2 units, whereas about 6.8% (95% CI; 5.2% to 8.8%) required surgery.[11]

CAUSES OF LOWER GASTROINTESTINAL BLEEDING

The causes of LGIB vary significantly based on the age at presentation; for example, among those less than 60 years of age, the leading causes of LGIB include colitis (infective, ischemic, inflammatory bowel disease, or an undetermined cause) as well as benign anorectal disorders (hemorrhoids, anal fissures, solitary rectal ulcer syndrome). In contrast, among patients more than 60 years of age, the leading cause is diverticular disease. Some of the most common causes of LGIB include diverticulosis, ischemic colitis, hemorrhoids, colorectal polyps or neoplasms, angioectasias, postpolypectomy bleeding, and inflammatory bowel disease.[4,12] A more complete list of causes of LGIB is shown in **Table 1**. Interestingly, it has been reported that in up to 25% of cases of LGIB, no cause can be documented.[10]

Table 1
Some causes of lower gastrointestinal bleeding

Category	Examples
Benign causes	Diverticular disease Hemorrhoids Angiodysplasia Anal fissure Solitary rectal ulcer Rectal prolapse Rectal varices
Colitis	Inflammatory bowel disease Ischemic colitis Infective colitis Undetermined colitis
Malignancy	Colon cancer Rectal cancer Anal cancer Metastatic or direct invasion from other primaries
Polyps	Adenomas Hamartomas
Vasculitis	Connective tissue diseases
Drug induced	Warfarin Aspirin Clopidogrel Direct oral anticoagulants Heparin
Iatrogenic	Postpolypectomy Endoscopic mucosal resection Endoscopic mucosal dissection Trauma Postoperative
Miscellaneous	Chronic anastomotic ulcer Hereditary hemorrhagic telangiectasia Arterio-enteric fistula Arteriovenous malformation Dieulafoy lesion Radiation proctitis

Data form Gralnek IM, Neeman Z, Strate LL. Acute lower gastrointestinal bleeding. N Engl J Med 2017;376:1054–63; and Strate LL, Ayanian JZ, Kotler G, et al. Risk factors for mortality in lower intestinal bleeding. Clin Gastroenterol Hepatol 2008;6:1004–10 [quiz: 955-].

CLINICAL PRESENTATION

The clinical presentation in LGIB varies depending on patient age at presentation as well as associated comorbidities. For example, a young man with bleeding hemorrhoids would usually only present with hematochezia. In contrast, an elderly man receiving antiplatelet and anticoagulation therapy who is bleeding following a polypectomy might present with brisk hematochezia, dizziness, decreased level of consciousness, signs of hemodynamic instability, decreased urine output, or hypovolemic shock. In general, hemodynamic instability is a rare presentation (2.3%) of LGIB.[10] Importantly, hemodynamic instability might indicate an upper gastrointestinal source of bleeding, which is found in about 15% of patients who present with suspected LGIB[13]; such a proximal cause can be suspected when patients have a prior history of upper gastrointestinal bleeding or in those receiving antiplatelet agents and/or anticoagulants.

HISTORY AND PHYSICAL EXAMINATION

Pertinent elements of the history include patients' comorbidities as well as medications, as these bear direct implications with regard to management and outcomes. Such clinical clues include the amount and frequency of bleeding, the color of stools (proximal vs distal source), as well as any accompanying abdominal pain. Painless rectal bleeding is more suggestive of diverticular or hemorrhoidal bleeding, whereas the presence of abdominal cramps associated with the subsequent passage of bloody diarrhea in patients with risk factors for cardiovascular disease might favor an ischemic cause. Alternately, bloody diarrhea of a short duration could be due to an infectious cause or inflammatory bowel disease.

The physical examination of patients, in addition to the initial assessment of level of consciousness, should include recording of vital signs, postural changes in pulse and blood pressure, assessment of cardiovascular and abdominal systems, and digital rectal examination. Examples of pertinent findings are signs of chronic liver disease that might point to a variceal cause of bleeding,[14] whereas (in rare cases) telangiectasia found in the mouth, ears, nose, hands, and/or feet might represent hereditary hemorrhagic telangiectasia.[15] Physical examination findings can at times potentially narrow down the differential diagnosis for the cause of bleeding.

Although not part of the physical examination, anoscopy might be of value to exclude regional causes of LGIB, principally actively bleeding hemorrhoids.

Some of the physical examination findings that should be sought when evaluating patients with LGIB are listed in **Table 2**.

Table 2
Some abnormal physical examination findings that might be found in patients with lower gastrointestinal bleeding

System	Finding
General examination	Confusion
	Cold clammy skin
	Poor capillary filling
	Skin telangiectasia
	Finds suggestive of neoplasia (cachexia, muscle wasting, lymphadenopathy, and so forth)
	Finds suggestive of liver cirrhosis or portal hypertension (gynecomastia, hair loss, wasting and so forth)
Vital signs	Tachycardia
	Hypotension
	Orthostatic changes
Abdominal examination	Abdominal tenderness
	Abdominal mass
	Splenomegaly
	Ascites
Rectal examination	Black stool (melena)
	Maroon-colored stool or fresh blood or clots (hematochezia)

Data from Refs.[17,20–22,24]

LABORATORY EVALUATION

The laboratory evaluation should include a complete blood count, serum electrolytes, blood urea nitrogen (BUN), creatinine, international normalized ratio (INR), and activated partial thromboplastin time. Blood grouping and a crossmatch for packed red blood cells should also be requested at the time of initial assessment. An elevated BUN might suggest an upper gastrointestinal bleeding source.[16]

Some of the laboratory investigations that have been associated with adverse outcomes are listed in **Table 3**.

RISK STRATIFICATION MODELS

Although most patients presenting with LGIB stop hemorrhaging on their own with conservative management only, there still remains a considerable associated risk of morbidity and mortality, especially in high-risk individuals and in those with multiple comorbidities.[17] Information gathering required for appropriate risk stratification of patients with LGIB requires obtaining a focused history, physical examination, and laboratory tests while simultaneously initiating resuscitation.

Risk stratification of patients presenting with presumptive LGIB aids in the appropriate triage of patients into different groups: those who can be managed on an outpatient basis with an electively scheduled endoscopy, patients who need to be monitored in a hospital setting versus those who need continuous monitoring in an ICU, some of whom in both cases may require a colonoscopy within the first 24 hours of presentation.

Several prognostication models have been developed[18–24]; some include clinical demographic characteristics as well as the presence or absence of comorbid conditions and findings on physical examination. Others also incorporate initial laboratory investigations and findings on reassessment after presentation.

A common feature of all of these stratification models is that they are usually derived from a small number of patients and lack validation in other populations limiting their generalizability and, possibly, their applicability. Furthermore, the end points used to identify such predictive models vary between studies. For example, there exists no unified definition of the composite outcome of severe bleeding that has been used in several of these predictive scores. The use of varying end points or definitions, therefore, further limits comparative analysis of prognostic properties.

Whether such patient stratification results in improved clinical outcomes or optimizing health care resource utilization has yet to be convincingly proven, as most scales have not been prospectively assessed let alone evaluated as formal

---

Table 3
Some laboratory investigations that are requested and possible results found in patients with lower gastrointestinal bleeding

Laboratory Test	Value Associated with Adverse Events
Hemoglobin or hematocrit	Decreased (<35% or 30%)
Platelet count	Decreased
Creatinine	Elevated (>133 mmol/L)
Blood urea nitrogen	Elevated
Prothrombin time	Elevated (1.2 control)
Albumin	Decreased (<3.0 g/dL)

Data from Refs.[21,22,24]

management intervention in high-quality studies. Some of the more commonly reported prognostic models are shown in **Table 4**. Most predictive tools have attempted to predict rebleeding, surgery, mortality, severe bleeding, adverse events, and the need for treatment (as opposed to conservative management) (**Table 5**).

Variables that have been associated with an increased 30-day mortality include age, dementia, metastatic cancer, chronic kidney disease, chronic pulmonary disease, anticoagulation use, admission hematocrit, and albumin[19](**Table 6**).

INITIAL HEMODYNAMIC RESUSCITATION

During the initial clinical assessment, 2 peripheral large-bore intravenous lines should be inserted. Intravenous fluids resuscitation using crystalloids should be initiated, especially in those with hemodynamic instability. Most of the recommendations in the literature as well as the recent guidelines addressing the management of LGIB[6] with regard to fluid resuscitation rely on data extrapolated either from the upper gastrointestinal bleeding or critical care literature. There are no clear recommendations based on good-quality evidence that address the volume, type, rates, or targets for fluid resuscitation nor blood transfusion targets in the specific population of LGIB.

With these limitations in mind, patients with LGIB should be resuscitated with crystalloids with the aim of normalizing the heart rate and blood pressure. As patients are usually older with multiple comorbidities, it is essential that the volume and rate of resuscitation be assessed frequently by bedside monitoring of volume status, avoiding volume overload.

If despite resuscitation efforts patients remain unstable or patients continue to bleed, early angiographic intervention should be considered. (See Kendall R. Beck and Amandeep K. Shergill's article, "Colonoscopy in Acute Lower Gastrointestinal Bleeding: Diagnosis, Timing, and Bowel Preparation"; and See Roy Soetikno and colleagues' article, "The Role of Endoscopic Hemostasis Therapy in Acute Lower Gastrointestinal Hemorrhage," in this issue.)

BLOOD AND BLOOD PRODUCT TRANSFUSION

A restrictive blood transfusion strategy has been associated with mortality and morbidity benefits in patients with upper gastrointestinal bleeding. In a meta-analysis that included 5 randomized controlled trials (RCTs) (4 published and 1 unpublished), a restrictive blood transfusion strategy, targeting a hemoglobin transfusion threshold of 7 to 8 g/dL aiming for 9 to 10 g/dL, was associated with a lower risk of all-cause mortality relative risk (RR): 0.65 (95% CI; 0.44–0.97) as well as a lower rebleeding rate: RR 0.58 (95% CI; 0.40–0.84).[25]

It should be noted that in patients with massive gastrointestinal bleeding, those with ischemic heart disease or cerebrovascular disease, a higher transfusion threshold value of 9 or 10 g/dL should be adopted. Although these data were generated in and are specific for upper gastrointestinal bleeding, it is reasonable to extrapolate these findings to patients with LGIB until appropriate information is reported.

A systematic review that included 4 RCTs as well as 6 cohort studies, none of which were specific for gastrointestinal bleeding (and all with significant methodological limitations), assessed platelet transfusion.[26] Based principally on expert opinion, when patients present with severe bleeding or when urgent endoscopic hemostasis is required, platelet transfusion should be considered when the platelet count is less than 50×10^9/L to maintain a target reaching that level. In some clinical settings, such as postcardiopulmonary bypass surgery, or in hemodialysis patients (clinical

Table 4
Some risk stratification scores used in lower gastrointestinal bleeding

Scoring System	Components	Cutoffs	Points	Comments
Kollef et al,[18] 1997 [ongoing **B**leeding, **L**ow systolic blood pressure, **E**levated prothrombin time, **E**rratic mental status, unstable comorbid **D**isease (**BLEED**)]	• Ongoing bleeding • Low SBP • Elevated prothrombin time • Erratic mental status • Unstable comorbid disease	NA SBP <100 mm Hg >1.2 control NA NA	NA	• The presence of any criteria at initial assessment in the emergency department would classify patients as high risk. • All other patients are classified as low risk. • It is used in both acute upper gastrointestinal bleeding or LGIB.

Sengupta & Tapper,[19] 2017	• Age
	
	• Dementia
	• Chronic kidney disease
	• Metastatic cancer
	• Systemic anticoagulant use
	• Chronic pulmonary disease
	• Admission hematocrit
	
	• Admission albumin
		<30
		30–39
		40–49
		50–59
		60–69
		70–79
		80–90
		>90
		NA
		
		<20
		20–29
		30–39
		>40
		<2
		2.0–2.9
		3.0–3.9
		>4
			−2
			−1
			0
			1
			2
			3
			4
			5
			5
			2
			
			5
			1
			
			2
			
			3
			1
			0
			−1
			13
			7
			0
			−7
				• The total score range is as follows: −10 to 36
				  Quartile 1: −10 to 1
				  Quartile 2: 2–4
				  Quartile 3: 5–8
				  Quartile 4: 9–36
				• The 30-d mortality was as follows:
				  Quartile 1: 3.6%–4.4%
				  Quartile 2: 4.9%–7.3%
				  Quartile 3: 9.9%–9.1%
				  Quartile 4: 24%–26%

Strate et al,[20] 2005	• HR • SBP • Nontender abdomen • Bleeding in first 4 h of presentation • Aspirin use • >2 Comorbid conditions (Charlson Index)	>100 bpm <115 mm Hg NA	NA	The risk groups are as follows: • Low (no risk factors) • Moderate (1–3 risk factors) • High (>3 risk factors) Severe bleeding is defined as follows: • Transfusion of ≥2 units of red blood cells • A decrease in hematocrit of ≥20% in the first 24 • Recurrent rectal bleeding after 24 h of stability (accompanied by a further decrease in hematocrit of ≥20%, and/or additional blood transfusions, and/or readmission for acute LGIB within 1 wk of discharge)

(continued on next page)

Table 4
(continued)

Scoring System	Components	Cutoffs	Points	Comments
Velayos et al,[21] 2004	• Initial hematocrit • Abnormal vital signs 1 h after initial medical evaluation • Gross blood on initial rectal examination	≤35% SBP <100 mm Hg or heart rate >100/min If present	NA	These are predictors of severe LGIB Severe LGIB, was defined as gross blood per rectum after leaving the emergency department is associated with either abnormal vital signs (SBP <100 mm Hg or HR >100/min) or more than a 2-unit blood transfusion during the hospitalization.
Das et al,[22] 2003	• Age • Sex • Cardiovascular disease • Chronic obstructive pulmonary disease • Chronic renal failure • Diabetes mellitus • Dementia • Cancer • Chronic liver disease • Colonic diverticulosis or its complications • Colonic arterio-vascular malformations • Use of nonsteroidal antiinflammatory drugs or anticoagulants • Alcoholism or smoking • Residence in a nursing home • Hematochezia • Orthostatic symptoms • Low SBP • Orthostatic signs • Change in mental status • White blood cell count • Packed-cell volume • Platelet count • Blood urea nitrogen • Creatinine • Activated partial thromboplastin time • Prothrombin time	NA <100 mm Hg NA	NA	The model was developed using an artificial neural network. It has a good negative predictive value (98%–100%); it may have a role in identifying patients who are at low risk of adverse outcomes.

(continued on next page)

Table 4
(continued)

Scoring System	Components	Cutoffs	Points	Comments
Newman et al,[23] 2012	• Hematocrit • Bright-red rectal bleeding • Age	<0.35 NA >60 y	—	Predictors for severe LGIB
Aoki et al,[24] 2016 (NOBLADS)	• NSAIDs use • No diarrhea • No abdominal tenderness • Blood pressure • Antiplatelet drugs use (nonaspirin) • Albumin level • >2 Comorbid conditions (Charlson Index) • Syncope	NA <100 mm Hg NA <3.0 g/dL NA 	1 1 1 1 1 1 1 1	The score discriminated patients requiring blood transfusion, a longer hospital stay, and intervention. • The percentage of patients who developed severe LGIB is as follows: Score 0 = 2.0% Score 1 = 10.0% Score 2 = 18.3% Score 3 = 34.8% Score 4 = 51.6% Score >5 = 75.7%

Abbreviations: bpm, beats per minute; HR, heart rate; NA, not applicable; NSAIDs, nonsteroidal antiinflammatory drugs; SBP, systolic blood pressure.

contexts that are associated with platelet dysfunction), or central nervous system trauma, a target of 100×10^9/L has been proposed.[26]

WHO SHOULD UNDERGO AN URGENT COLONOSCOPY?

Using the aforementioned risk stratification models, patients with high-risk features or those who have evidence of ongoing bleeding should undergo an urgent colonoscopy within 24 hours of presentation.[6] In a case-control study looking at those patients with diverticular bleeding undergoing a colonoscopy and endoscopic hemostasis for stigmata of hemorrhage within 6 to 12 hours after a polyethylene glycol (PEG) solution preparation, the associated risk of bleeding and surgery was reduced.[27] Of note, this was an observational study and included only a small number of patients. Two RCTs demonstrated that a colonoscopy performed in less than 12 hours after a rapid PEG preparation resulted more often in a definitive diagnosis compared with those who had an elective procedure (odds ratio 2.6 [95% CI; 1.1–6.2]) but did not affect any other outcomes.[13,28] Observational data suggest that an earlier colonoscopy is associated with reduced hospital length of stay.[29]

WHO CAN HAVE A COLONOSCOPY ON A NONURGENT BASIS?

In patients with no high-risk features and for those who are at high risk and do not have signs of active bleeding, a colonoscopy can be deferred to the next available elective timeslot, after an adequate PEG purge has been administered.

PERIPROCEDURAL MANAGEMENT OF ANTIPLATELET AND ANTICOAGULATION THERAPY

The incidence of LGIB in patients receiving low-dose aspirin (ASA) ranges from 0.48 to 0.74 cases per 1000 person-years.[30] In one study, the use of ASA was

Table 5
Variables associated with various outcomes based on numerous studies

	Outcomes					
	Rebleeding	Surgery	Mortality	Severe Bleeding	Adverse Events	Need for Treatment
History						
Age >60 y	—	—	—	Yes	Yes	—
Male sex	Yes	—	Yes	—	—	Yes
Unstable comorbid illness	Yes	Yes	Yes	—	—	—
>2 comorbid conditions[a]	Yes	—	—	Yes	—	—
Smoking	—	—	—	—	Yes	—
Aspirin use	Yes	—	—	Yes	—	—
Antiplatelet agent	—	—	—	Yes	—	—
NSAID use	—	—	—	Yes	—	—
Syncope	Yes	—	—	Yes	—	—
No diarrhea	—	—	—	Yes	—	—
History of colon diverticulosis or angiodysplasia	Yes	—	Yes	—	—	Yes
History of bright red blood per rectum	Yes	—	Yes	Yes	—	Yes
Physical examination						
SBP<100 mm Hg	Yes	Yes	Yes	Yes	—	Yes
SBP<115 mm Hg	Yes	—	—	Yes	—	—
HR >100 bpm	Yes	—	—	Yes	—	—
Abnormal hemodynamic parameters	—	—	—	—	Yes	—
Abnormal vital signs after 1 h	—	—	—	Yes	Yes	—
Altered mental status	Yes	Yes	Yes	—	—	—
Nontender abdomen	Yes	—	—	Yes	—	—
Gross blood on initial rectal examination	—	—	—	Yes	Yes	—
Hospital course						
Bleeding in first 4 h of presentation	Yes	—	—	Yes	—	—
Continuing hemorrhage	Yes	Yes	Yes	—	—	—
Rebleeding	—	—	—	—	Yes	—
Laboratory values	—	—	—	—	—	—
Hematocrit <35% or 30%	Yes	—	Yes	Yes	Yes	Yes
Prothrombin time >1.2 control	Yes	Yes	Yes	—	—	—
High creatinine (>133 mmol/L)	Yes	—	Yes	—	Yes	Yes
Albumin <3.0 g/dL	—	—	—	Yes	—	—

Abbreviations: bpm, beats per minute; HR, heart rate; NSAID, nonsteroidal antiinflammatory drug; SBP, systolic blood pressure.

[a] The following are based on the Charlson Index: (1) The study by Kollef and colleagues[18] included patients with both upper gastrointestinal bleeding and LGIB. (2) Das and coolleagues[22] developed an artificial neural network to classify patients according to each outcome.

Data from Refs.[18,20–24,42]

Table 6
Predictors of 30-day mortality

Variable	Odds Ratio	95% Confidence Interval
Age	1.02	1.00–1.03
Dementia	5.24	1.63–14.27
Metastatic cancer	4.95	3.18–7.71
Chronic kidney disease	2.20	1.45–3.34
Chronic pulmonary disease	1.64	1.05–2.53
Use of anticoagulants	1.47	0.94–2.25
Admission hematocrit	0.98	0.95–1.01
Admission albumin	0.35	0.25–0.47

Data from Sengupta N, Tapper EB. Derivation and internal validation of a clinical prediction tool for 30-day mortality in lower gastrointestinal bleeding. Am J Med 2017;130:601.e1–8.

associated with an adjusted RR of 2.7 (95% CI; 1.8–4.1), whereas that associated with non-ASA antiplatelet agents was 1.8 (95% CI; 1.0–2.0).[31] Thus, in conjunction with fluid resuscitation and blood transfusion, if needed, patients who are receiving antiplatelet therapies or anticoagulants should have their risk profile appropriately reviewed and the benefits and limitations of continuing or withholding these medications determined. As part of the periprocedural management of LGIB, low-dose ASA should be withheld in cases of primary prophylaxis; if used in secondary prophylaxis, ASA should be continued without interruption.[4,6] In patients with LGIB receiving dual antiplatelet therapy (DAPT), the non-ASA antiplatelet agent should be temporarily withheld for no more than 7 days, whereas ASA is continued without interruption. If LGIB has occurred in the 30 days after coronary stent insertion or 90 days after an acute coronary syndrome, DAPT should not be interrupted because of the mortality associated with acute stent thrombosis.[6] These recommendations are often updated by specialty societies, and the reader is cautioned to stay up to date with such changes or consult with an expert colleague at the time of acute management.

Patients receiving anticoagulants are at an increased risk of developing LGIB, RR of 5.4 (95% CI; 3.0–9.7).[31] Although the data are limited, when comparing vitamin K antagonists with direct oral anticoagulants (DOACs), both exhibited similar risks of LGIB (1%), RR of 0.88 (95% CI; 0.67–1.15).[32]

Some of the risk factors that have been associated with an increased risk of gastrointestinal bleeding while on anticoagulation (both vitamin K antagonists and DOACs) include older age (>75 years), renal impairment, prior history of gastrointestinal bleeding, use of ASA, use of nonsteroidal antiinflammatory drugs, and heart failure.[33] Although an elevated INR is associated with increased rebleeding, as well as a greater need for surgery and mortality, these might reflect observed associations rather than demonstrating actual causal relationships. An INR level between 1.5 and 2.5 should not delay endoscopic intervention and possible hemostasis (based on data from the upper gastrointestinal bleeding literature[34]). Reversal agents should be given before endoscopic intervention if the INR is greater than 2.5.[6]

In a propensity-matched cohort study of a large Japanese database, the risk of adverse events in the periprocedural period were higher among patients who used warfarin plus heparin bridging versus DOACs plus heparin bridging;[35] the worsened outcomes included postprocedural bleeding, thromboembolism, and in-hospital death. Although the study covered a wide range of endoscopic interventions and was not specific to LGIB, it does question the practice of bridging with heparin in patients on anticoagulation therapy. No recommendations about bridging in the context of acute LGIB or upper gastrointestinal bleeding were made in the most recent guidelines from the American College of Gastroenterology, the American Society for Gastrointestinal Endoscopy, or the European Society of Gastrointestinal Endoscopy.[5,6,36]

Although these are general recommendations, each case should ideally be managed with consultation with an internist, hematologist, and/or cardiologist.

A general outline of the initial management of patients with acute LGIB is shown in **Fig. 1**.

ORAL INTAKE

Patients are usually kept fasting and as soon as permissible, for patients requiring early colonoscopy, a bowel preparation solution is administered in view of early colonoscopy in the form of at least 4 L of a PEG solution over 3 to 4 hours. Patients are permitted to take clear liquids up to 2 hours before the procedure.[4] Although the insertion of a nasogastric tube in suspected cases of upper gastrointestinal bleeding has fallen out of favor,[37] it might be used in this setting for the subsequent administration of bowel preparation solutions in those who cannot tolerate it orally (up to 33%), provided the aspiration risk is low.

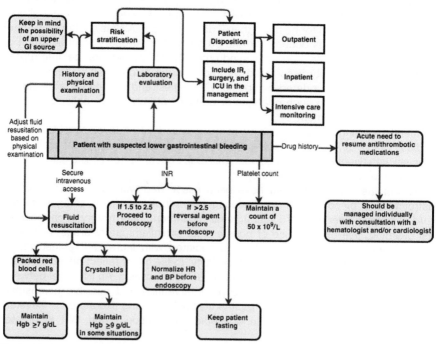

Fig. 1. The various aspects of caring for patients with acute lower gastrointestinal bleeding. BP, blood pressure; GI, gastrointestinal; Hgb, hemoglobin; HR, heart rate; ICU, intensive care unit; IR, interventional radiology.

INITIAL MANAGEMENT PERSPECTIVE IN VIEW OF SUBSEQUENT SECONDARY PROPHYLAXIS

Recurrent bleeding after a single episode of LGIB varies depending on the cause; in a single-center study 47% of patients with proven diverticular bleeding had recurrent bleeding after a median time of 8.1 months.[38] Although for angioectasias, a small RCT estimated that the rate of recurrent bleeding in the placebo arm at 1 year was 45% and reached 64% at 2 years.[39] Contrary to upper gastrointestinal bleeding, no study has assessed the acute discontinuation followed by early versus later reintroduction of ASA in LGIB (the former approach was favored in upper gastrointestinal bleeding based on one RCT[40]).

After an episode of LGIB, approaches to avoid recurrent bleeding include stopping non-ASA nonsteroidal antiinflammatory drugs, especially in those with a prior history of bleeding from diverticulosis or angioectasias,[6] as these have been proven to be associated with recurrent LGIB.[41] Here to, as mentioned for acute management, ASA should be avoided when it is used as a primary prophylaxis; but when used as secondary prophylaxis it should not be interrupted, especially in patients who are at high risk of adverse cardiovascular outcomes.[6]

SUMMARY

LGIB is associated with significant mortality and morbidity and has not been well studied with regard to specific hemodynamic resuscitation recommendations. Appropriate management depends on proper risk stratification with simultaneous resuscitation while optimization of underlying comorbidities. Preparation toward early colonoscopy (within the 24 hours following presentation) should be considered in patients at high risk of negative outcomes stable enough to undergo this procedure.

REFERENCES

1. Peery AF, Crockett SD, Barritt AS, et al. Burden of gastrointestinal, liver, and pancreatic diseases in the United States. Gastroenterology 2015;149: 1731–41.e3.
2. Ell C, May A. Mid-gastrointestinal bleeding: capsule endoscopy and push-and-pull enteroscopy give rise to a new medical term. Endoscopy 2006;38:73–5.
3. Raju GS, Gerson L, Das A, et al, American Gastroenterological Association. American Gastroenterological Association (AGA) Institute technical review on obscure gastrointestinal bleeding. Gastroenterology 2007;133:1697–717.
4. Gralnek IM, Neeman Z, Strate LL. Acute lower gastrointestinal bleeding. N Engl J Med 2017;376:1054–63.
5. ASGE Standards of Practice Committee, Pasha SF, Shergill A, Acosta RD, et al. The role of endoscopy in the patient with lower GI bleeding. Gastrointest Endosc 2014;79:875–85.
6. Strate LL, Gralnek IM. ACG clinical guideline: management of patients with acute lower gastrointestinal bleeding. Am J Gastroenterol 2016;111:755.
7. Laine L, Yang H, Chang SC, et al. Trends for incidence of hospitalization and death due to GI complications in the United States from 2001 to 2009. Am J Gastroenterol 2012;107:1190–5 [quiz: 6].
8. Lanas A, Garcia-Rodriguez LA, Polo-Tomas M, et al. Time trends and impact of upper and lower gastrointestinal bleeding and perforation in clinical practice. Am J Gastroenterol 2009;104:1633–41.

9. Tinegate H, Pendry K, Murphy M, et al. Where do all the red blood cells (RBCs) go? Results of a survey of RBC use in England and North Wales in 2014. Transfusion 2016;56:139–45.

10. Oakland K, Guy R, Uberoi R, et al. Acute lower GI bleeding in the UK: patient characteristics, interventions and outcomes in the first nationwide audit. Gut 2018;67(4):654–62.

11. Roshan Afshar I, Sadr MS, Strate LL, et al. The role of early colonoscopy in patients presenting with acute lower gastrointestinal bleeding – a systematic review and meta-analysis. Therap Adv Gastroenterol 2018;11. 1756283X18757184.

12. Almadi MA, Almessabi A, Wong P, et al. Ectopic varices. Gastrointest Endosc 2011;74:380–8.

13. Laine L, Shah A. Randomized trial of urgent vs. elective colonoscopy in patients hospitalized with lower GI bleeding. Am J Gastroenterol 2010;105:2636–41 [quiz: 42].

14. Alharbi A, Almadi M, Barkun A, et al. Predictors of a variceal source among patients presenting with upper gastrointestinal bleeding. Can J Gastroenterol 2012; 26:187–92.

15. Thrash B, Patel M, Shah KR, et al. Cutaneous manifestations of gastrointestinal disease: part II. J Am Acad Dermatol 2013;68:211.e1-33 [quiz: 44–46].

16. Al-Naamani K, Alzadjali N, Barkun AN, et al. Does blood urea nitrogen level predict severity and high-risk endoscopic lesions in patients with nonvariceal upper gastrointestinal bleeding? Can J Gastroenterol 2008;22:399–403.

17. Strate LL, Ayanian JZ, Kotler G, et al. Risk factors for mortality in lower intestinal bleeding. Clin Gastroenterol Hepatol 2008;6:1004–10 [quiz: 955-].

18. Kollef MH, O'Brien JD, Zuckerman GR, et al. BLEED: a classification tool to predict outcomes in patients with acute upper and lower gastrointestinal hemorrhage. Crit Care Med 1997;25:1125–32.

19. Sengupta N, Tapper EB. Derivation and internal validation of a clinical prediction tool for 30-day mortality in lower gastrointestinal bleeding. Am J Med 2017;130: 601.e1-e8.

20. Strate LL, Saltzman JR, Ookubo R, et al. Validation of a clinical prediction rule for severe acute lower intestinal bleeding. Am J Gastroenterol 2005;100:1821–7.

21. Velayos FS, Williamson A, Sousa KH, et al. Early predictors of severe lower gastrointestinal bleeding and adverse outcomes: a prospective study. Clin Gastroenterol Hepatol 2004;2:485–90.

22. Das A, Ben-Menachem T, Cooper GS, et al. Prediction of outcome in acute lower-gastrointestinal haemorrhage based on an artificial neural network: internal and external validation of a predictive model. Lancet 2003;362:1261–6.

23. Newman J, Fitzgerald JE, Gupta S, et al. Outcome predictors in acute surgical admissions for lower gastrointestinal bleeding. Colorectal Dis 2012;14:1020–6.

24. Aoki T, Nagata N, Shimbo T, et al. Development and validation of a risk scoring system for severe acute lower gastrointestinal bleeding. Clin Gastroenterol Hepatol 2016;14:1562–70.e2.

25. Odutayo A, Desborough MJ, Trivella M, et al. Restrictive versus liberal blood transfusion for gastrointestinal bleeding: a systematic review and meta-analysis of randomised controlled trials. Lancet Gastroenterol Hepatol 2017;2:354–60.

26. Razzaghi A, Barkun AN. Platelet transfusion threshold in patients with upper gastrointestinal bleeding: a systematic review. J Clin Gastroenterol 2012;46: 482–6.

27. Jensen DM, Machicado GA, Jutabha R, et al. Urgent colonoscopy for the diagnosis and treatment of severe diverticular hemorrhage. N Engl J Med 2000; 342:78–82.
28. Green BT, Rockey DC, Portwood G, et al. Urgent colonoscopy for evaluation and management of acute lower gastrointestinal hemorrhage: a randomized controlled trial. Am J Gastroenterol 2005;100:2395–402.
29. Navaneethan U, Njei B, Venkatesh PG, et al. Timing of colonoscopy and outcomes in patients with lower GI bleeding: a nationwide population-based study. Gastrointest Endosc 2014;79:297–306.e12.
30. Garcia Rodriguez LA, Martin-Perez M, Hennekens CH, et al. Bleeding risk with long-term low-dose aspirin: a systematic review of observational studies. PLoS One 2016;11:e0160046.
31. Lanas A, Carrera-Lasfuentes P, Arguedas Y, et al. Risk of upper and lower gastrointestinal bleeding in patients taking nonsteroidal anti-inflammatory drugs, antiplatelet agents, or anticoagulants. Clin Gastroenterol Hepatol 2015;13: 906–12.e2.
32. Miller CS, Dorreen A, Martel M, et al. Risk of gastrointestinal bleeding in patients taking non-vitamin k antagonist oral anticoagulants: a systematic review and meta-analysis. Clin Gastroenterol Hepatol 2017;15(11):1674–83.e3.
33. Lanas-Gimeno A, Lanas A. Risk of gastrointestinal bleeding during anticoagulant treatment. Expert Opin Drug Saf 2017;16:673–85.
34. Barkun AN, Bardou M, Kuipers EJ, et al. International consensus recommendations on the management of patients with nonvariceal upper gastrointestinal bleeding. Ann Intern Med 2010;152:101–13.
35. Nagata N, Yasunaga H, Matsui H, et al. Therapeutic endoscopy-related GI bleeding and thromboembolic events in patients using warfarin or direct oral anticoagulants: results from a large nationwide database analysis. Gut 2017 [pii:-gutjnl-2017-313999][Epub ahead of print].
36. Gralnek IM, Dumonceau JM, Kuipers EJ, et al. Diagnosis and management of nonvariceal upper gastrointestinal hemorrhage: European Society of Gastrointestinal Endoscopy (ESGE) guideline. Endoscopy 2015;47:a1–46.
37. Dakik HK, Srygley FD, Chiu ST, et al. Clinical performance of prediction rules and nasogastric lavage for the evaluation of upper gastrointestinal bleeding: a retrospective observational study. Gastroenterol Res Pract 2017;2017:3171697.
38. Aytac E, Stocchi L, Gorgun E, et al. Risk of recurrence and long-term outcomes after colonic diverticular bleeding. Int J Colorectal Dis 2014;29:373–8.
39. Swanson E, Mahgoub A, MacDonald R, et al. Medical and endoscopic therapies for angiodysplasia and gastric antral vascular ectasia: a systematic review. Clin Gastroenterol Hepatol 2014;12:571–82.
40. Sung JJ, Lau JY, Ching JY, et al. Continuation of low-dose aspirin therapy in peptic ulcer bleeding: a randomized trial. Ann Intern Med 2010;152:1–9.
41. Nagata N, Niikura R, Aoki T, et al. Impact of discontinuing non-steroidal antiinflammatory drugs on long-term recurrence in colonic diverticular bleeding. World J Gastroenterol 2015;21:1292–8.
42. Strate LL, Orav EJ, Syngal S. Early predictors of severity in acute lower intestinal tract bleeding. Arch Intern Med 2003;163:838–43.

Colonoscopy in Acute Lower Gastrointestinal Bleeding
Diagnosis, Timing, and Bowel Preparation

Kendall R. Beck, MD[a], Amandeep K. Shergill, MD[b,c],*

KEYWORDS

- Bowel preparation • Hemorrhage • Length of stay • Review • Hematochezia
- Nuclear scintigraphy • CT angiography

KEY POINTS

- Urgent upper endoscopy should be the initial test in a patient with hemodynamically unstable hematochezia or if the source cannot be localized to the lower gastrointestinal tract.
- Colonoscopy after rapid colon purge should be the initial diagnostic and therapeutic modality used in patients with suspected acute lower gastrointestinal bleeding.
- Early colonoscopy is safe, has the potential to diagnose and treat nearly any lesion causing lower gastrointestinal bleeding, and may decrease the duration of stay.
- More research is needed to determine the true effect of early colonoscopy on clinically meaningful outcomes in patients presenting with lower gastrointestinal bleeding.

INTRODUCTION

Acute lower gastrointestinal (GI) bleeding (LGIB) is a common cause of hospitalization, and frequently leads to morbidity in the United States and worldwide.[1] Although the mortality rate is generally low (<5%), advanced age, intestinal ischemia, and comorbid illness portend a higher risk of death.[2] In the United States, the incidence of LGIB ranges from 20.5 to 27 per 100,000 persons per year with a greater than 200-fold increase from the third to the ninth decades of life.[1] The increasing incidence with age may be related to comorbid disease and associated polypharmacy, including the increasing use of aspirin, nonsteroidal antiinflammatory drugs, and anticoagulants.[3]

Disclosures: A.K. Shergill is the recipient of a Pentax research gift for ergonomics.
[a] UCSF Division of Gastroenterology, Department of Medicine, University of California San Francisco, 1701 Divisadero Street, Suite 120, San Francisco, CA 94115, USA; [b] Department of Medicine, University of California San Francisco, 505 Parnassus Avenue S-357, San Francisco, CA 94143, USA; [c] Department of Medicine, San Francisco Veteran's Affairs Hospital, 4150 Clement Street, VA 111B/GI Section, San Francisco, CA 94121, USA
* Corresponding author. San Francisco Veteran's Affairs Hospital, 4150 Clement Street, VA 111B/GI Section, San Francisco, CA 94121.
E-mail address: amandeep.shergill@ucsf.edu

In addition, GI-specific illnesses prevalent in the elderly may predispose to LGIB, such as diverticulosis, arteriovenous malformation, and colonic neoplasm.[4] Clinical features associated with a worse outcome in LGIB include hemodynamic instability at presentation, comorbid illnesses, age greater than 60 years, a history of diverticulosis or angioectasia, an elevated creatinine, and anemia (initial hematocrit of $\leq$35%) on presentation.[5] Presentation ranges from a small amount of rectal bleeding to episodes of massive hematochezia with passage of blood clots.

Many aspects regarding the care of patients experiencing LGIB are extrapolated from upper GI bleeding (UGIB) guidelines, such as blood transfusion strategies.[6] However, there is a small but growing body of literature to guide the care of these patients, particularly regarding the role of colonoscopy. Colonoscopy is considered the initial test of choice for most patients presenting with LGIB given its diagnostic capabilities, therapeutic potential, and relative safety,[5] although optimal timing is not well-defined in the literature. This review examines the role of colonoscopy in the diagnosis of acute LGIB, including the timing of colonoscopy and recommendations for colon preparation in the setting of acute LGIB.

DIAGNOSIS

The most common causes of acute LGIB include diverticulosis, ischemia, hemorrhoids, neoplasm, angioectasias, postpolypectomy bleeding, inflammatory bowel disease, and infectious colitis (**Fig. 1**). Less common causes include stercoral ulcer, colorectal varices, radiation proctitis, nonsteroidal antiinflammatory drug–induced

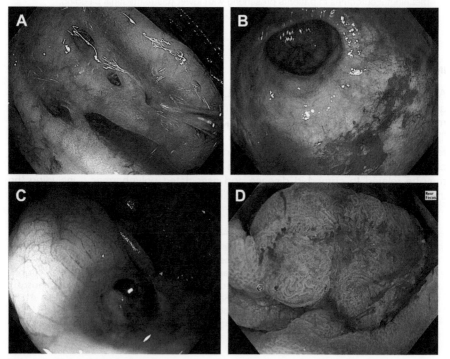

Fig. 1. Findings on colonoscopy. (*A*) Active diverticular hemorrhage. (*B*) Bleeding arteriovenous malformation. (*C*) Postpolypectomy ulcer with visible vessel. (*D*) Bleeding colonic polyp.

colopathy, and Dieulafoy lesion.[6] When a patient is admitted to the hospital with an acute LGIB, they may first require hemodynamic stabilization. Once stabilized, a thorough history and physical examination should be performed in an attempt to grade the severity and identify the location of bleeding as upper GI tract, the small intestine, or the large intestine,[5] and to guide further management. It is important to note that 11% to 15%[7,8] of patients presenting with hematochezia suspicious for an LGIB will in fact be experiencing an upper GI bleed. If the patient is hemodynamically unstable, an urgent upper endoscopy should be the initial test to rule out an upper intestinal source of bleeding.[9] Although a nasogastric tube can be used to evaluate for an upper GI source,[5] it is most helpful if it is positive for a bloody aspirate, which, in 1 retrospective cohort study, was associated with a likelihood ratio of 11 (95% confidence interval [CI], 4–30) for an upper gastrointestinal source of bleeding.[10] In the prospective, randomized controlled trial (RCT) by Laine and Shah,[8] 15% of enrolled patients with clinically significant hematochezia were ultimately diagnosed with an upper GI source of bleeding, despite a negative nasogastric aspirate. The authors of that study advocate for considering upper endoscopy before colonoscopy in all patients presenting with clinically significant hematochezia.[8]

If an upper GI source of bleeding is considered clinically unlikely, the nasogastric tube can be left in place to facilitate preparation for colonoscopy, required by 33% of patients presenting with acute LGIB in 1 prospective study.[7] Adequate bowel preparation is critical to the technical success of colonoscopy, because colonoscopy has the ability to detect and treat bleeding lesions, and to prevent recurrent bleeding in lesions with high-risk stigmata.

COLON PREPARATION

It is of paramount importance to achieve an adequate preparation of the colon when performing colonoscopy for LGIB, because mucosal-based lesions may be easily missed in a poorly prepped colon and the risk of perforation is likely lower in a well-prepped colon.[5] In general, studies of urgent colonoscopy in acute LGIB have used large volume (4-6 L) polyethylene glycol (PEG)-based preparations administered over a 3- to 4-hour timeframe[5,7] and are clinically referred to as a "rapid purge." The stool should be checked frequently during preparation, and PEG should be provided until the patient has achieved an adequate preparation. To facilitate the rapid purge,[11] a nasogastric tube should only be used in patients at low risk for aspiration.[5]

There are few data on the adequacy of bowel preparation in the setting of acute LGIB. One of the earliest studies of the safety and efficacy of colonoscopy after PEG preparation for acute hematochezia included 35 patients. The authors reported excellent mucosal visualization, identified colonic bleeding lesions in 24 of 35 patients, and bleeding sources proximal to the ileocecal valve in 3 of 35. The per-oral preparation was well-tolerated, and there were no adverse events from the preparation or the colonoscopy, suggesting that PEG preparation in this setting is both safe and effective for cleansing the colon.[12] In prospective trials evaluating urgent colonoscopy with PEG preparation, PEG preparation of 4 to 6 L taken over 3 to 4 hours seems to achieve adequate visualization in approximately 90% of cases. In the RCT by Laine and Shah,[8] patients received 4 L of PEG solution over 3 hours for urgent colonoscopy performed within 12 hours of presentation, and although bowel prep quality was not reported, only 7% of patients required repeat colonoscopies owing to inadequate preparation. In the RCT by Green and colleagues,[13] patients received 4 to 6 L of PEG over 3 to 4 hours with a colonoscopy performed within 2 hours of clearance of stool and clots, and in this study only 8% of patients in the urgent colonoscopy group had a poor prep.

The American College of Gastroenterology recommends against performing unprepared colonoscopy in patients with acute LGIB.[5] A study by Repaka and colleagues[14] evaluated the feasibility of performing immediate unprepared hydroflush colonoscopy in patients presenting with severe LGIB. The study included only 13 procedures, and patients were given a tap water enema followed by immediate colonoscopy, without oral bowel preparation. The cecal intubation rate was low at 69.2%, and a definite source of bleeding was only found in 38.5% of patients, with 25% of patients experiencing recurrent bleeding during the same hospitalization.

There are few studies evaluating factors that predict inadequate bowel preparation in the hospitalized patient with acute LGIB. Predictors of poor preparation identified in the outpatient setting have been extrapolated to the inpatient setting, and these are listed in **Box 1**.[5,15] Simply being hospitalized is 1 predictor of inadequate bowel preparation and, thus, inpatients often require more than the traditional 4 L of PEG.

The safety of bowel preparation in patients with acute LGIB has not been extensively studied, but overall, bowel preparation is thought to be safe. Niikura and colleagues[16] evaluated the safety of preparation and colonoscopy in 161 patients hospitalized for acute LGIB compared with 161 control patients without signs of GI bleeding undergoing elective colonoscopy. Sixteen (9%) patients with LGIB experienced an adverse event during preparation (7% developed hypotension, and 2% experienced vomiting), and no significant difference was found between patients with LGIB and controls. None of the patients experienced volume overload, aspiration pneumonia, or loss of consciousness. Aspiration precautions are recommended in older and debilitated patients.[5]

TIMING OF COLONOSCOPY

The optimal timing of colonoscopy in the setting of acute LGIB continues to be debated. The definition of urgent colonoscopy used within the literature generally

---

Box 1
Predictors of poor preparation

Cirrhosis

Complex medical history (as measured by higher American Society of Anesthesiologists class, or ≥8 medical prescriptions)

Constipation

Higher body mass index

Medications, particularly the use of narcotics and tricyclic antidepressants

Neurologic conditions (eg, a history of Parkinson's disease, spinal cord injury, stroke, or dementia)

Older age

Presence of diabetes

Prior gastrointestinal surgical resection

Procedure time

Only those that are likely to relate to hospitalized patients are included.
Data from Strate LL, Gralnek IM. ACG clinical guideline: management of patients with acute lower gastrointestinal bleeding. Am J Gastroenterol 2016;111(4):459–74; and Ness RM, Manam R, Hoen H, et al. Predictors of inadequate bowel preparation for colonoscopy. Am J Gastroenterol 2001;96(6):1797–802.

refers to a colonoscopy performed within 6 to 24 hours of presentation,[13,17–21] with a more stringent definition of 6 to 12 hours used in the prospective trials published to date.[7,8,13] The rationale behind the performance of earlier colonoscopy for LGIB is driven by the same principles of early endoscopy for upper GI bleeding: diagnosing and treating a bleeding source. However, performance of colonoscopy requires a bowel preparation and lesion identification is potentially more difficult in the colon. Thus, the diagnostic and therapeutic yield of early colonoscopy and its effect on patient-related outcomes such as transfusion requirements, need for surgery, and duration of stay are important considerations that many studies of various designs have attempted to address.

In general, studies evaluating the use of urgent colonoscopy versus elective colonoscopy or radiographic procedures have been plagued by insufficient statistical power related to low sample sizes, relatively rare events (ie, low mortality rates in LGIB), or inherent biases related to retrospective design, nonblinding, or local practices. Attempts at metaanalysis have been limited by heterogeneity of the data, making it difficult to draw conclusions regarding the benefit of urgent colonoscopy in patients presenting with acute LGIB. These methodologic issues are further confounded by the natural history of LGIB, whereby approximately 70% of patients stop bleeding spontaneously.[8] Nevertheless, most major societies recommend early colonoscopy[5,9] because the diagnostic yield of colonoscopy ranges from 45% to 90%.[5] Metaanalyses demonstrate that earlier colonoscopy seems to be associated with higher detection of bleeding lesions, stigmata of recent hemorrhage and/or therapeutic interventions.[20–22] However, there seems to be no significant change in the duration of stay, rebleeding, transfusion requirement, or surgery in patients undergoing early versus elective colonoscopy. A summary of the studies evaluating optimal timing of colonoscopy is included in **Table 1**.

Initial retrospective studies suggested a high diagnostic yield and decreased duration of stay with early colonoscopy.[17,18] Strate and Syngal[17] evaluated the timing of colonoscopy and duration of stay in 252 patients hospitalized with acute LGIB, of whom 57% (144) underwent inpatient colonoscopy. They found that colonoscopy revealed the source of bleeding in 89% of examinations, and that time to colonoscopy was an independent predictor of hospital duration of stay (hazard ratio of 2.02 for a shorter stay; 95% CI, 1.5–2.6; $P<.0001$). The absence of visible blood or active bleeding at colonoscopy was also an independent predictor of a shorter duration of stay. The authors concluded that the identification of low-risk lesions during colonoscopy likely resulted in earlier discharge, because patients with less severe bleeding who did not undergo colonoscopy stayed in the hospital longer than those undergoing colonoscopy in less than 12 hours, and for about the same amount of time as those undergoing colonoscopy between 12 and 24 hours.[17]

Prospective studies have demonstrated mixed results of early colonoscopy on duration of stay and diagnostic yield. One of the first was a paired prospective study conducted by Jensen and colleagues[7] that enrolled 121 patients with severe hematochezia and diverticulosis and performed urgent colonoscopy (within 6–12 h) after rapid purge with 5 to 6 L of PEG solution within 1 hour of clearance of stool. In the first part of the study, 73 patients who underwent diagnostic only colonoscopy with medical and surgical treatment were compared with 48 patients in the second part of the study who underwent therapeutic colonoscopy if a source of bleeding was found. Definite/presumed diverticular hemorrhage was found in 23% and 0% in the diagnostic only colonoscopy group versus 21% and 29% in the therapeutic colonoscopy group. Of the patients with definite diverticular hemorrhage, patients who underwent endoscopic therapy had significantly lower rebleeding rates (0% vs 53%; $P = .005$), need for emergency hemicolectomy (0% vs 35%; $P = .03$), and decreased hospital

Table 1
Comparison of studies evaluating timing of colonoscopy

Study and Date	Study Type	Timing of Urgent Colonoscopy	Diagnostic Yield for Colonoscopy	Clinically Important Outcomes	Negative Outcomes
Tada et al,[33] 1991	Retrospective	3 d	89.3% if performed within 3 d; 68.5% if performed after 4 d of presentation	No difference in diagnostic yield if colonoscopy performed within 3 d	Accuracy decreased if performed after 3 d
Strate & Syngal,[17] 2003	Retrospective	48 h	Early colonoscopy improved diagnostic yield	Time to colonoscopy predicted duration of stay (HR 2.02)	Identifying a diagnosis and the use of endoscopic therapy not associated with duration of stay
Nathan Schmulewitz et al,[18] 2003	Retrospective	24 h	88.9%	Early colonoscopy led to reduced duration of stay	Hemodynamic instability, higher comorbidity, tagged red blood cell scan, and need for surgery associated with less likelihood of discharge
Green et al,[13] 2005	RCT	8 h	42%	Improved diagnostic yield vs standard care (42% vs 22%)	No difference in duration of stay, ICU stay, transfusion, rebleeding and need for surgery
Laine & Shah[8] 2010	RCT	6–15 h	78% urgent, 67% elective	Nonsignificant trend toward shorter duration of stay in urgent group	No difference in bleeding, transfusion, hospitalization cost
Navaneethan et al,[19] 2014	Population based	<24 h	Not reported	Shorter duration of stay, cost, blood transfusion	No difference in mortality
Seth et al,[23] 2017	Metaanalysis	8–24 h	No difference between urgent and elective	Increased detection of stigmata of hemorrhage (OR, 2.85; 95% CI, 1.90–4.28)	No difference in rebleeding, need for surgery, or mortality
Kouanda et al,[24] 2017	Metaanalysis	8–4 h	No difference between urgent and elective	Increased use of endoscopic intervention	No difference in duration of stay or cost
Sengupta et al,[22] 2017	Metaanalysis	<24 h	Detection of bleeding source (OR, 2.97; 95% CI, 2.11–4.19) higher with early colonoscopy	Likelihood of endoscopic intervention (OR, 3.99; 95% CI, 2.59–6.13) higher with early colonoscopy	No difference in rebleeding, duration of stay, or surgery

Abbreviations: CI, confidence interval; HR, hazard ratio; ICU, intensive care unit; OR, odds ratio; RCT, randomized controlled clinical trial.

duration of stay (median of 2 days vs 5 days; $P<.001$).[7] In the first RCT by Green and colleagues,[13] urgent purge preparation followed by colonoscopy within 8 hours of presentation was compared with their standard care algorithm, which was based on a red blood cell nuclear scintigraphy scan followed by angiographic intervention versus elective colonoscopy in those with negative scans (typically occurred within 4 days of admission). Urgent colonoscopy allowed for a definite diagnosis of the source of bleeding more often than the standard care group (42% vs 22%; odds ratio, 2.6; 95% CI, 1.1–6.2), although the absolute numbers were small (13 of 50 vs 8 of 50, respectively). There was no difference in other important outcomes including mortality, duration of stay, intensive care unit stay, transfusion requirements, rebleeding, and surgery. A second RCT by Laine and Shah[8] enrolled 85 patients with severe intestinal bleeding. Esophagogastroduodenoscopy was performed within 6 hours of presentation and before randomization, and identified 15% with an upper GI bleeding source despite having a negative nasogastric aspirate. The remaining 72 patients were randomized to urgent (purge preparation with 4 L of PEG over 3 hours, followed by colonoscopy within 12 hours of presentation) or elective colonoscopy (36 in each group). They found no difference in clinical outcomes such as further bleeding, transfusion, duration of stay, subsequent interventions, or hospital costs between the 2 groups. They did see a trend toward shorter hospitalization in the urgent colonoscopy arm in those without further bleeding, but this study was terminated early owing to logistical issues that negatively affected patient enrollment. Thus, an effect of a shorter duration of stay might not be realized without an adequate sample size.

To address the sample size problem, Navaneethan and colleagues[19] used the Nationwide Inpatient Sample, an administrative dataset, to conduct a nationwide population-based study evaluating in-hospital mortality, duration of stay, and hospitalization costs in patients who underwent early (<24 hours) or delayed (>24 hours) colonoscopy. Of 58,296 patients discharged with LGIB, 22,720 (38.9%) had a colonoscopy performed during that hospitalization and 9156 (40.1%) underwent early colonoscopy. Patients who underwent early colonoscopy had a shorter duration of stay (2.9 days vs 4.6 days; $P<.001$), decreased need for blood transfusion (44.6% vs 53.8%; $P<.001$), and lower hospitalization costs ($22,142 vs $28,749; $P<.001$). There was no difference in mortality.

Three recently published systematic reviews with metaanalysis attempted to address the question of whether urgent colonoscopy improves outcomes in LGIB. Seth and colleagues[23] evaluated 6 studies (2 RCT and 4 observational), including 23,419 patients undergoing either urgent or elective colonoscopy. Urgent colonoscopy was performed within 8 to 24 hours of presentation with lower GI bleeding. There was an increased rate of detection of stigmata of recent hemorrhage in those undergoing urgent colonoscopy; however, this did not translate into reduced rebleeding, mortality, or need for surgery. Kouanda and colleagues[24] evaluated 12 studies with 10,172 patients in the urgent colonoscopy arm, and 14,224 in the elective arm. Urgent colonoscopy was performed within 8 to 24 hours of presentation with lower GI bleeding. They found an increase in the use of endoscopic therapeutic interventions in patients undergoing urgent colonoscopy, but this also did not translate into improved clinically relevant outcomes such as bleeding source localization, adverse event rates, rebleeding rates, transfusion requirement, hospitalization costs, or mortality. One reason they may have found a difference in the use of endoscopic therapies was that hemorrhoidal band ligation was included as an intervention. Although there was a trend toward a decreased duration of stay, this was not statistically significant.[24] The third metaanalysis was conducted by Sengupta and colleagues,[22] and included 6 studies with a total of 422 patients in the early (<24 hours) colonoscopy arm and 479 in the delayed (>24 hours) colonoscopy arm. No statistically significant difference was seen in transfusion requirements, need for surgery, or in-hospital mortality between the groups. Early colonoscopy was associated with a higher rate of detecting a definite source of bleeding (odds ratio, 2.97; 95% CI, 2.11–4.19) and with the performance of an endoscopic intervention (odds ratio, 3.99; 95% CI, 2.59–6.13).

Despite the lack of a clear benefit of early colonoscopy for reducing the duration of stay, transfusion requirements or need for surgery, given the relatively good accuracy of colonoscopy to detect and potentially treat the majority of the causes that contribute to LGIB, the major society guidelines recommend that colonoscopy be the initial diagnostic procedure for patients presenting with acute LGIB.[5,9] The 2016 American College of Gastroenterology guidelines suggest that colonoscopy be performed within 24 hours of presentation with hematochezia in patients with high-risk clinical features or signs of ongoing bleeding. Patients without signs of active bleeding and without high-risk clinical features can be performed at the next available time slot.[5] The American Society of Gastrointestinal Endoscopy defines early colonoscopy as occurring between 8 and 24 hours. These guidelines suggest that patients presenting with severe hematochezia and hemodynamic instability should undergo upper endoscopy followed by colonoscopy if negative. If patients are hemodynamically stable, then a colonoscopy can be performed first, followed by upper endoscopy if negative.[9]

Technical Aspects

A colonoscope with a working channel of at least 3.3 mm is preferred for adequate irrigation and suctioning capabilities and to allow for the passage of large size hemostasis tools (10-F).[5] The terminal ileum should be intubated to ensure the bleeding is not the result of a small bowel source. A water jet pump can facilitate evaluation of the colonic mucosa by irrigating and dislodging residual stool, blood, and clots.[5] The use of a distal attachment cap can facilitate inspection of potential bleeding sources, particularly in the case of suspected diverticular bleed. In a retrospective study of diverticular bleeding, the site of bleeding was within the dome of the diverticulum in approximately one-third of cases, which can be difficult to adequately visualize.[25] The cap can be used to evert the diverticulum with gentle suctioning to allow for complete evaluation of a diverticulum for endoscopic stigmata[26] that might otherwise be missed. Endoscopic therapeutic modalities will be discussed later in this issue.

Safety

Colonoscopy is safe in the acute LGIB population, with estimates of adverse events within the literature ranging from 0.3% to 1.3%.[7,13,18,27] Although colonoscopy is overall considered a safe procedure, patients who are acutely ill may be at a higher risk for adverse events.[28,29] Potential adverse events of colonoscopy include abdominal pain, bowel perforation, worsened bleeding, septicemia, and complications related to sedation, including cardiopulmonary events.[30] Adverse events of elective colonoscopy are increased in elderly patients, particularly octogenarians,[31] and these data are extrapolated to urgent colonoscopy. This finding is particularly relevant to the LGIB population given that elderly patients are overrepresented in this group. Congestive heart failure, electrolyte abnormalities, and aspiration are potential risks related to rapid purge preparation.[27,32]

Radiographic Diagnostic Modalities

Radiographic modalities are alternatives to colonoscopy for the diagnosis, and in the case of angiography, management of LGIB. A summary of clinically important differences between colonoscopy and radiographic modalities is provided in **Table 2**.

Table 2
Comparison of colonoscopy versus radiographic diagnostic modalities in acute lower gastrointestinal bleeding

Diagnostic Modality	Diagnosis (%)	Bleeding Rate Required	Sedation Required	Colon Preparation	Advantages
Colonoscopy[32,34–36]	74–100	No bleeding	Usually	Yes	Diagnose lesion, perform therapeutic maneuver
Tagged RBC[32,37,38]	40–73	0.1–0.35 mL/min	No	No	Identify intermittent bleeding
MDCT[20,39–41]	24–94	0.3 mL/min	No	No	High accuracy
Angiography[21,42–44]	23–72	0.5–1 mL/min	Yes	No	Perform therapeutic maneuver

Abbreviations: Tagged RBC, red blood cell nuclear scintigraphy; MDCT, multidetector row computed tomography.

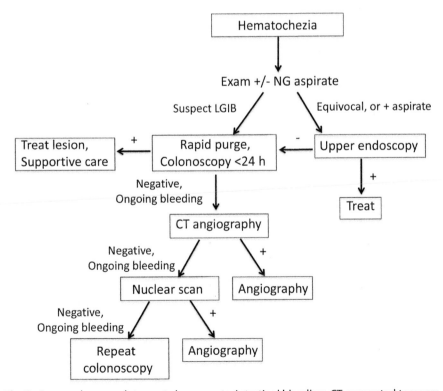

Fig. 2. Proposed approach to acute lower gastrointestinal bleeding. CT, computed tomography; NG, nasogastric.

The 2016 American College of Gastroenterology guidelines suggest that colonoscopy performed within 24 hours of presentation is the initial test of choice in a patient experiencing an acute LGIB; however, radiographic interventions should be considered when high-risk patients with ongoing bleeding do not respond adequately to resuscitation, because they may not tolerate bowel preparation and colonoscopy.[5]

SUMMARY

We have summarized our approach to LGIB in **Fig. 2**. A detailed history, physical examination, and laboratory evaluation is performed on presentation. If an upper GI source of bleeding is deemed unlikely and the patient is hemodynamically stable, we recommend a rapid purge with 4 to 6 L of a PEG solution over 3 to 4 hours with the goal of clear effluent, followed by early colonoscopy timed to within 2 hours of clearance of stool and within 24 hours of presentation. If the patient is hemodynamically unstable, or an upper source of bleeding is not ruled out via history, physical, or nasogastric tube, then an urgent upper endoscopy is performed first. If esophagogastroduodenoscopy is negative, then the patient will undergo a colonoscopy. In patients whose bleeding seems to have spontaneously ceased and who can undergo nonurgent inpatient colonoscopy, bowel preparation is performed overnight or deferred to the next available examination. Radiographic modalities are reserved for patients who are too unstable to tolerate a colon preparation and colonoscopy or for those who have recurrent bleeding without a source diagnosed or managed by prior colonoscopy.

REFERENCES

1. Longstreth GF. Epidemiology and outcome of patients hospitalized with acute lower gastrointestinal hemorrhage: a population-based study. Am J Gastroenterol 1997;92(3):419–24.
2. Strate LL, Ayanian JZ, Kotler G, et al. Risk factors for mortality in lower intestinal bleeding. Clin Gastroenterol Hepatol 2008;6(9):1004–10.
3. Lanas A, Garcia-Rodriguez LA, Polo-Tomas M, et al. The changing face of hospitalisation due to gastrointestinal bleeding and perforation. Aliment Pharmacol Ther 2011;33(5):585–91.
4. James JJ, Farrell LS. Gastrointestinal bleeding in older people. Gastroenterol Clin North Am 2000;29(1):1–36.
5. Strate LL, Gralnek IM. ACG clinical guideline: management of patients with acute lower gastrointestinal bleeding. Am J Gastroenterol 2016;111(4):459–74.
6. Gralnek IM, Neeman Z, Strate LL. Acute lower gastrointestinal bleeding. N Engl J Med 2017;376(11):1054–63.
7. Jensen DM, Machicado GA, Jutabha R, et al. Urgent colonoscopy for the diagnosis and treatment of severe diverticular hemorrhage. N Engl J Med 2000; 342:78–82.
8. Laine L, Shah A. Randomized trial of urgent vs. elective colonoscopy in patients hospitalized with lower GI bleeding. Am J Gastroenterol 2010;105(12):2636–41 [quiz: 42].
9. ASGE Standard of Practice Committee, Pasha SF, Shergill A, et al. The role of endoscopy in the patient with lower GI bleeding. Gastrointest Endosc 2014; 79(6):875–85.
10. Witting MD, Magder L, Heins AE, et al. Usefulness and validity of diagnostic nasogastric aspiration in patients without hematemesis. Ann Emerg Med 2004; 43(4):525–32.

11. Wong Kee Song LM, Baron TH. Endoscopic management of acute lower gastro-intestinal bleeding. Am J Gastroenterol 2008;103(8):1881–7.

12. Caos A, Benner KG, Manier J, et al. Colonoscopy after Golytely preparation in acute rectal bleeding. J Clin Gastroenterol 1986;8(1):46–9.

13. Green BT, Rockey DC, Portwood G, et al. Urgent colonoscopy for evaluation and management of acute lower gastrointestinal hemorrhage: a randomized controlled trial. Am J Gastroenterol 2005;100(11):2395–402.

14. Repaka A, Atkinson MR, Faulx AL, et al. Immediate unprepared hydroflush colo-noscopy for severe lower GI bleeding: a feasibility study. Gastrointest Endosc 2012;76(2):367–73.

15. Ness RM, Manam R, Hoen H, et al. Predictors of inadequate bowel preparation for colonoscopy. Am J Gastroenterol 2001;96(6):1797–802.

16. Niikura R, Nagata N, Shimbo T, et al. Adverse events during bowel preparation and colonoscopy in patients with acute lower gastrointestinal bleeding compared with elective non-gastrointestinal bleeding. PLoS One 2015;10(9):e0138000.

17. Strate LL, Syngal S. Timing of colonoscopy impact on length of hospital stay in patients with acute lower intestinal bleeding. Am J Gastroenterol 2003;98(2):317–22.

18. Nathan Schmulewitz DAF, Rockey DC. Early colonoscopy for acute lower GI bleeding predicts shorter hospital stay: a retrospective study of experience in a single center. Gastrointest Endosc 2003;58(6):841–6.

19. Navaneethan U, Njei B, Venkatesh PG, et al. Timing of colonoscopy and out-comes in patients with lower GI bleeding: a nationwide population-based study. Gastrointest Endosc 2014;79(2):297–306.e12.

20. Rondonotti E, Marmo R, Petracchini M, et al. The American Society of Gastroen-terology (ASGE) diagnostic algorithm for obscure gastrointestinal bleeding- Eight burning questions from everyday clinical practice. Dig Liver Dis 2013;45(3):179–85.

21. Gary Zuckerman CP. Acute lower intestinal bleeding Part II: etiology, therapy, and outcomes.pdf. Gastrointest Endosc 1999;49(2):228–38.

22. Sengupta N, Tapper EB, Feuerstein JD. Early versus delayed colonoscopy in hos-pitalized patients with lower gastrointestinal bleeding: a meta-analysis. J Clin Gastroenterol 2017;51(4):352–9.

23. Seth A, Khan MA, Nollan R, et al. Does urgent colonoscopy improve outcomes in the management of lower gastrointestinal bleeding? Am J Med Sci 2017;353(3):298–306.

24. Kouanda AM, Somsouk M, Sewell JL, et al. Urgent colonoscopy in patients with lower GI bleeding: a systematic review and meta-analysis. Gastrointest Endosc 2017;86(1):107–17.e1.

25. Kaltenbach T, Watson R, Shah J, et al. Colonoscopy with clipping is useful in the diagnosis and treatment of diverticular bleeding. Clin Gastroenterol Hepatol 2012;10(2):131–7.

26. Sanchez-Yague A, Kaltenbach T, Yamamoto H, et al. The endoscopic cap that can (with videos). Gastrointest Endosc 2012;76(1):169–78.e1-2.

27. Gary R, Zuckerman CP. Acute lower intestinal bleeding Part 1:clinical presenta-tion and diagnosis. Gastrointest Endosc 1998;48(6):606–16.

28. Hokama A, Uehara T, Nakayoshi T, et al. Utility of endoscopic hemoclipping for colonic diverticular bleeding. Am J Gastroenterol 1997;92:543–6.

29. Zuccaro G. Management of the adult patient with acute lower gastrointestinal bleeding. Am J Gastroenterol 1998;93(8):1202–8.

30. ASGE Standards of Practice Committee, Fisher DA, Maple JT, et al. Complications of colonoscopy. Gastrointest Endosc 2011;74(4):745–52.
31. Day LW, Kwon A, Inadomi JM, et al. Adverse events in older patients undergoing colonoscopy: a systematic review and meta-analysis. Gastrointest Endosc 2011; 74(4):885–96.
32. Lhewa DY, Strate LL. Pros and cons of colonoscopy in management of acute lower gastrointestinal bleeding. World J Gastroenterol 2012;18(11):1185–90.
33. Tada M, Shimizu S, Kawai K. Emergency colonoscopy for the diagnosis of lower intestinal bleeding preparation. Gastroenterol Jpn 1991;26(3):121–4.
34. Jensen DM, Machicado GA. Diagnosis and treatment of severe hematochezia. Gastroenterology 1988;95(6):1569–74.
35. Lisa L, Strate SS. Predictors of utilization of early colonoscopy vs radiography for severe lower intestinal bleeding. Gastrointest Endosc 2005;61(1):46–52.
36. Strate LL, Naumann CR. The role of colonoscopy and radiological procedures in the management of acute lower intestinal bleeding. Clin Gastroenterol Hepatol 2010;8(4):333–43 [quiz: e44].
37. Ford PV, Bartold SP, Fink-Bennett DM, et al. Procedure guideline for gastrointestinal bleeding and Meckel's diverticulum scintigraphy. J Nucl Med 1999;40: 1226–32.
38. Lee SS, Oh TS, Kim HJ, et al. Obscure gastrointestinal bleeding: diagnostic performance of multidetector CT enterography. Radiology 2011;259(3):739–48.
39. Chua AE, Ridley LJ. Diagnostic accuracy of CT angiography in acute gastrointestinal bleeding. J Med Imaging Radiat Oncol 2008;52(4):333–8.
40. Garcia-Blazquez V, Vicente-Bartulos A, Olavarria-Delgado A, et al. Accuracy of CT angiography in the diagnosis of acute gastrointestinal bleeding: systematic review and meta-analysis. Eur Radiol 2013;23(5):1181–90.
41. Awais M, Haq TU, Rehman A, et al. Accuracy of 99mTechnetium-labeled RBC Scintigraphy and MDCT with gastrointestinal bleed protocol for detection and localization of source of acute lower gastrointestinal bleeding. J Clin Gastroenterol 2016;50(9):754–60.
42. Winzelberg GG, Froelich JW, McKusick KA, et al. Radionuclide localization of lower gastrointestinal hemorrhage. Radiology 1981;139:465–9.
43. Luc Defreyne MU, Vanlangenhove P, Van Maele G, et al. Angiography for acute lower gastrointestinal hemorrhage-efficacy of cut film compared with digital subtraction techniques. J Vasc Interv Radiol 2003;14(3):313–22.
44. William S, Yi GG, Sava JA. Localization and definitive control of lower gastrointestinal bleeding with angiography and embolization. Am Surg 2013;79:375–80.

The Role of Endoscopic Hemostasis Therapy in Acute Lower Gastrointestinal Hemorrhage

Roy Soetikno, MD, MS, MSM[a,b,]*, Naoki Ishii, MD[c],
Jennifer M. Kolb, MD[d], Hazem Hammad, MD[d],
Tonya Kaltenbach, MD, MS[e]

KEYWORDS

- Lower gastrointestinal bleeding • Endoscopic hemostasis • Endoscopic therapy
- Endoscopic clipping • Diverticulosis

KEY POINTS

- The authors stratify lower gastrointestinal bleeding (LGIB) patients with an on-going bright red blood per rectum, hemodynamic instability, syncope, history of aspirin or anticoagulant use, and/or 2 or more comorbidities but with nontender abdominal examination to have severe bleeding, then proceed with rapid bowel purge for urgent colonoscopy.
- The authors perform urgent colonoscopy after (1) the patient has been hemodynamically resuscitated, is clinically stable, and has completed a rapid bowel purge; and (2) the appropriate resources and equipment are made available at the bedside (scopes and accessories); and (3) an endoscopist with experience and skill in the treatment of LGIB is present at the bedside.
- The authors treat diverticular bleeding using endoscopic clipping directly when bleeding is from the neck of the diverticulum; using clipping or band ligation from within a cap when bleeding is from the dome; or, more recently, using the over-the-scope clip for bleeding from anywhere in a diverticulum.

Disclosures: Consultant for Olympus (R. Soetikno). Consultant for Medtronics (H. Hammad). Consultant for Olympus (T. Kaltenbach).
[a] Advanced GI Endoscopy, Mountain View, California, USA; [b] Department of Gastroenterology, University of Indonesia, Jakarta, Indonesia; [c] Division of Gastroenterology, Koga Hospital, Ibaraki, Japan; [d] Division of Gastroenterology, University of Colorado Anschutz Medical Center, Denver, CO, USA; [e] Clinical Medicine, University of California, San Francisco, Veterans Affairs San Francisco Medical Center, San Francisco, CA, USA
* Corresponding author. Advanced GI Endoscopy, University of Indonesia, Jakarta, Indonesia.
E-mail address: Soetikno@earthlink.net

Gastrointest Endoscopy Clin N Am 28 (2018) 391–408
https://doi.org/10.1016/j.giec.2018.02.010
1052-5157/18/© 2018 Elsevier Inc. All rights reserved.

There comes a time to every life when the past recedes and the future opens.
It's that moment when you turn to face the unknown.
Some will turn back to what they already know.
Some will walk straight ahead into uncertainty.
I can't tell you which one is right. But, I can tell you which one is more fun.
                                                        Philip H. Knight (1938–)

INTRODUCTION

The authors began to incorporate endoscopic hemostasis to treat acute lower gastro-intestinal bleeding (LGIB) into their practice in the late 1990s out of necessity. Patients with acute LGIB were predominantly elderly with significant morbidity and mortality. Interventional radiology and surgery pose high risk for morbidity and mortality.[1] At that time, the authors turned their faces to the unknown and walked straight into the uncertainty. The authors made emergency colonoscopy service available, and worked diligently to make it safe and effective by applying and adapting our therapeutic endoscopy knowledge to treat severe LGIB. As soon as they showed the potentials of endoscopy, which happened relatively quickly, their endoscopy service became the de facto primary diagnostic and therapeutic modality for acute LGIB. Along the way, they collected their experiences and shared them widely.[1–7]

Outcome data pertaining to the efficacy of endoscopic treatment in patients with LGIB is heterogeneous and sparse, although there is a growing recent literature, especially from our Japanese colleagues. Thus, the guidelines to manage patients with LGIB have been difficult to develop and are not yet robust.[8] Herein, based on available literature and the authors' 20-year experience, they summarized the role of endoscopic hemostasis therapy in acute severe LGIB with a focus on how to perform the hemostasis techniques.

DEFINITION AND CLASSIFICATION

LGIB is traditionally defined as bleeding that originates from a source distal to the ligament of Treitz to the anus. More recently, however, the definition has been changed to refer to bleeding originating between the ileocecal valve and the anus. Bleeding from a source between the ligament of Treitz and the ileocecal valve is defined as middle gastrointestinal (GI) bleeding.[9]

Patients with severe upper GI bleeding may be thought to have acute severe LGIB. In select cases with clinical presentation or risk factors for upper GI bleeding, placement of a nasogastric tube for aspiration of gastric and duodenal contents can be very useful. When the authors aspirate blood (old or fresh), they classify patients as having upper GI bleeding and, thus, pursue an emergency upper endoscopy. When they aspirate bile, the authors classify patients as having LGIB and proceed with preparation for colonoscopy.[10] In cases in which a colonic source of bleeding is not identified, they intubate the terminal ileum (**Fig. 1**) and, if still unrevealing, perform an upper endoscopy immediately. In essence, the possibility of an upper or a middle GI source is always considered in the management of acute severe LGIB, until a colonic source has been identified.

The stratification of the severity of LGIB is important to identify patients who may benefit from an urgent colonoscopy. In contrast to the Blatchford score,[11] which is used to stratify patients presenting with acute upper GI bleeding and aids in assessment to target high-risk patients who may benefit most from an emergency endoscopy, a well-validated scoring system to stratify patients with LGIB has not yet

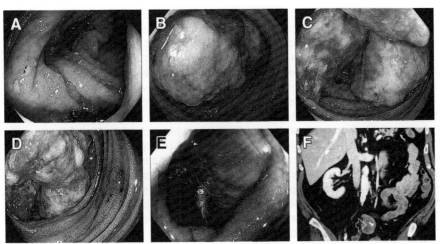

Fig. 1. A 71-year-old man presented with a 6-unit acute severe lower GI bleed. After stabilization, he underwent rapid bowel purge and colonoscopy. (*A*) There were scattered clots in the colon, particularly in the cecum. (*B*) On intubation of the terminal ileum and examination proximally, a large pigmented mass with exudate and vessels was seen. (*C*) It was obstructing the lumen, though with some maneuvering, the colonoscope could traverse the mass. (*D*) The patient had a history of mediastinal metastatic melanoma of unknown primary site, and the authors thus interpreted the mass appearance as melanoma. They tattooed the mucosa at the same level as the mass, and (*E*) placed an endoscopic clip for marking. (*F*) CT shows the ileal mass with the clip (*arrow*) close by (*arrow*). The India ink can serve as a marker in case resection is needed. The clip can assist the interventional radiologist in case the patient needs a selective embolization. The clip can also help the surgeon to plan where to perform the surgical incision.

been developed. Thus, at present, the authors stratify LGIB patients in two categories. The first is severe bleeding; these are patients with an on-going bright red blood per rectum, hemodynamic instability, syncope, history of aspirin or anticoagulant use, or two or more comorbidities but with non-tender abdominal examination.[12] In these patients, they proceed with immediate bowel preparation and emergent colonoscopy.[13] The second is stratified as less severe LGIB. Patients with less severe LGIB are scheduled to have elective colonoscopy, unless bleeding recurs, in which case the will perform the procedure urgently. Note that an urgent colonoscopy, performed within 24 hours of admission, should be performed only if it is safe and feasible to do in relation to the patient's overall condition after hemodynamic resuscitation, availability of resources, and (of equal importance) endoscopic expertise.[8]

PATIENT PREPARATION

Bowel preparation is critical to performing a safe and effective urgent colonoscopy. Invariably, it is required that the bowel is evacuated of stool, blood clots, and fresh blood. The key is to initiate the bowel preparation as soon as possible and to administer it as a rapid bowel purge.[14] Following hemodynamic stabilization, the authors prepare patients for their urgent colonoscopy by using a rapid bowel purge. In a rapid purge, they use 4 to 6 L of polyethylene glycol given over 2 to 3 hours. They prescribe metoclopramide 10 mg if the patient develops nausea and administer the solution via a nasogastric tube, if necessary.[15] Other endoscopists have used intravenous erythromycin as a promotility agent. If there is concern for large-residual contents or need for deep sedation to reduce the risk of aspiration, nasogastric suction should be done immediately before colonoscopy. Patients with known bowel obstruction or gastroparesis should not receive rapid preparation.

In patients presenting with postpolypectomy bleeding, the authors also administer bowel preparation to remove large blood clots and bile, unless they develop the bleeding before they leave the endoscopy unit or before they have received solid food.

The authors perform urgent colonoscopy when the patient has had nothing by mouth for 2 hours and, ideally, within 2 hours of completion of the bowel purge. However, in patients who continue to pass fresh blood per rectum, they perform the colonoscopy sooner. In such cases, to reduce the risk of aspiration, they explain to the patients that they will perform the procedure without sedation. Other endoscopists have reported performing colonoscopy without bowel preparation in patients who were unstable and undergoing intravenous fluid resuscitation.[16] They, however, restricted the procedure to be performed only by an expert colonoscopist with experience in performing an unprepped colonoscopy. Unprepped colonoscopy is not recommended by recent LGIB guidelines.[13]

CLINICAL PRESENTATION AND DIFFERENTIAL DIAGNOSES

The differential diagnoses of acute severe LGIB are broad, including diverticular bleeding; angiodysplasia; ischemia; radiation proctopathy; infectious, inflammatory, hemorrhoids; and Dieulafoy bleeding. Clues from the patient presentation can help narrow the differential diagnosis, and facilitate the appropriate diagnostic and management strategy.

Diverticular bleeding is the most common cause of acute LGIB, especially in adults older than 60 years with comorbidities. It presents as acute, painless, bright red blood per rectum that is generally self-limited. The presence of colonic diverticula identified on cross-sectional imaging or on previous colonoscopy, along with a personal history of diverticular bleeding, point to this as the most likely cause of LGIB.

Angiodysplasia is especially prevalent in elderly patients with cardiovascular disease or chronic renal failure, and is typically located in the cecum and ascending colon in Western populations versus the left colon in Asian populations.[17] Angiodysplasia can present as severe or occult LGIB.

Ischemic colitis is the likely cause of LGIB in patients who have recently sustained hypotension or hemodynamic shock, although in some the episodes were not obvious (**Fig. 2**).

History of bright red blood on wiping or that fills the toilet bowl only with bowel movements is suggestive of hemorrhoidal bleeding. It can cause severe bleeding, although this presentation is uncommon.

In patients who have received abdominal radiation for previous malignancies, radiation proctopathy should be suspected. Meanwhile, LGIB in patients who describe weight loss, change in bowel habits, obstructive symptoms, or family history of GI malignancies raise concern for colorectal cancer. In a younger, otherwise healthy patient, infectious and inflammatory causes should be considered first. Abdominal pain, bloody diarrhea, and fever warrant evaluation for inflammatory bowel disease, in which bleeding would be more likely with ulcerative colitis than Crohn's disease.

ENDOSCOPIC TECHNIQUES

Various techniques are useful to treat severe LGIB; the choice depends on the cause and the availability of expertise. Additionally, because LGIB is not as

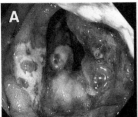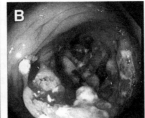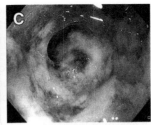

Fig. 2. LGIB from ischemic colitis. (*A*) An otherwise healthy 71-year-old gentleman presented with nausea or vomiting and syncope followed by hematochezia. Endoscopic examination revealed diffuse severe inflammation from the hepatic flexure to the ascending colon. Biopsies were consistent with ischemic colitis. (*B*) Friable mucosa with deep ulcerations. No endoscopic intervention was done and the bleeding resolved with supportive care. (*C*) In another case, an elderly woman presented with complete heart block and hypotension. Soon after she developed bloody diarrhea. Sigmoidoscopy showed a diffuse area of circumferential severely congested, inflamed, dusky mucosa at 30 cm proximal to the anus.

common as acute upper GI bleeding, some accessories required may not be available; therefore, the choice of technique also depends on the availability of accessories. To streamline and standardize accessories, the authors have primarily focused on endoscopic clipping to treat a variety of LGIB. In addition to clipping, the authors have used argon plasma coagulation (APC) to treat arteriovenous malformations (AVMs) and banding to treat hemorrhoids. However, in their unit in the United States, they do not regularly have the band ligation device that is suitable for colonoscope length. The authors do not use simple epinephrine injection by itself because of its limited efficacy. They refrain from using monopolar thermocoagulation given its risk of causing perforation in the colon.

ENDOSCOPIST, ENDOSCOPE, AND ENDOSCOPE ACCESSORIES SELECTION
Endoscopist Selection

Colonoscopy in patients with severe LGIB can be quite challenging. The patient may be quasi stable. The lumen may be filled with blood clots or fresh blood. Some bowel prep may still be in the colon and mixed with the blood. Visualization may be reduced because blood absorbs the light of the colonoscope. In addition, because diverticular disease is the most common cause of severe LGIB, many patients have a narrowed left colon and many diverticular openings. Multiple insertions of the colonoscope may be necessary. Therefore, colonoscopy during severe LGIB is not appropriate for a beginner trainee to perform. In these cases, the trainee can learn more by observing and assisting the attending who performs the procedure.

Endoscope and Endoscope Accessories Selection

The authors typically use an adult colonoscope with water jet to be able to suction the clots and fluids. Carbon dioxide, rather than air, is the standard insufflation medium. Water immersion technique is not used. In fact, a major limitation of water immersion insertion technique is that it cannot be used in the treatment of LGIB because visualization is impaired by blood.

In severe LGIB cases, the authors often will need to perform multiple insertions. The first insertion is to determine the type and source of bleeding. During insertion, the colon is washed and suctioned as much as possible to identify the source. If the cause is found to be nondiverticular, treatment is performed. If diverticular bleeding stigmata are found at the neck, then direct clipping is applied. If diverticular bleeding stigmata are found at the dome, then a clip is placed near its opening to mark it, and the colonoscope is withdrawn. The second insertion is performed after the colonoscope has been equipped with either a banding accessory or a distal attachment cap. The bleeding diverticulum is then banded or clipped from within a cap.

If only nonbleeding diverticula were found, then the colonoscope can be withdrawn and equipped with a cap. In these cases, the purpose of the second insertion is to investigate the diverticula and to determine which has bled (**Fig. 3**).

Of note, the authors use the therapeutic upper endoscope in the management of bleeding from the left colon because it is more flexible than the adult colonoscope.[3] Owing to its large working channel and its ability to retroflex within a smaller radius than the colonoscope, this endoscope can also be used for bleeding from the anorectum.[4]

Marking of the diverticulum with bleeding stigmata is critical to maintain orientation.[18] Intermittent bleeding and colonoscope inadvertent movements can cause a

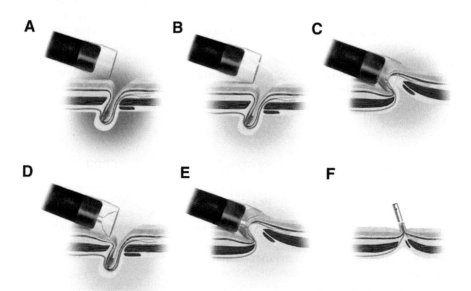

Fig. 3. Schematic of using an endoscopic cap to diagnose diverticular bleeding and to treat it using an endoscopic clip. (*A*) The endoscope was fitted with a distal attachment cap. (*B*) Blood from the lumen and diverticulum was washed using a foot-pedal controlled water jet and suctioned away. (*C*) The cap was useful to visualize diverticula that are located behind folds. More importantly, gentle suctioning of the diverticulum into the cap causes it to evert, thus allowing examination of its dome. (*D*) After the bleeding vessel was identified, an endoscopic clip was loaded into the working channel of the endoscope and placed within the cap. (*E*) The diverticulum was everted into the cap with the aim to place the bleeding vessel precisely into an awaiting clip. (*F*) The bleeding vessel was successfully clipped. This technique is best performed using endoscopic clips that can be partially opened, opened and closed, and rotated. (*From* Kaltenbach T, Watson R, Shah J, et al. Colonoscopy with clipping is useful in the diagnosis and treatment of diverticular bleeding. Clin Gastroenterol Hepatol 2012;10(2):133; with permission.)

surgeon to easily lose track of the culprit diverticulum. In addition, bleeding may become more profuse and interventional radiology may become necessary. In such cases, the metal clip will provide locational guidance to the radiologist.

TECHNIQUE FOR SPECIFIC DISEASE
Diverticular Bleeding

Diagnosis
Diverticular bleeding is the most common cause of acute severe LGIB. Although most (approximately 80%) diverticular bleeding is self-limited, it is important to understand and recognize the diverticular bleeding stigmata (**Fig. 4**) because some patients can develop massive bleeding that requires endoscopic management. Bleeding can occur at the neck or along the dome of the diverticula from an injured branch of the submucosal plexus of vessels, which originate from a sizable submucosal artery (**Fig. 5**). As such, the endoscopic stigmata of recent bleeding from the diverticulum may be immediately visible when at the neck or may need to be exposed by inverting the diverticula when located at the dome. Using a clear plastic cap with gentle suction, the diverticulum can be inverted. Depending on the size of the diverticulum, the exposed cap length may need to be adjusted (**Fig. 6**). The water jet is critical to provide optimal visualization to clear clot or debris from the culprit diverticulum and delineate the bleeding stigmata.

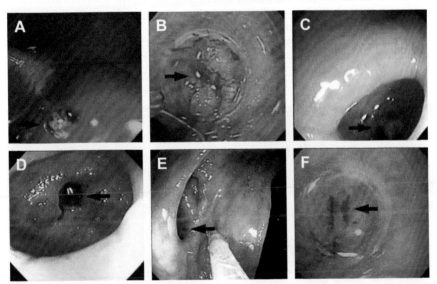

Fig. 4. Stigmata of diverticular bleeding (*arrow*). (*A*) A clot was seen at the neck of the diverticulum with an actively bleeding vessel. (*B*) Use of a distal attachment cap to evert the diverticulum reveals an actively bleeding small vessel at the dome of the diverticulum. (*C*) A visible vessel was seen at the dome of the diverticulum without active bleeding. (*D*) A clot was visualized at the dome of the diverticulum. (*E*) A pigmented spot was seen at the neck of the diverticulum, suggestive of recent bleeding. (*F*) A small erosion was seen at the neck of the diverticulum suggestive of recent bleeding. (*From* Kaltenbach T, Watson R, Shah J, et al. Colonoscopy with clipping is useful in the diagnosis and treatment of diverticular bleeding. Clin Gastroenterol Hepatol 2012;10(2):132; with permission.)

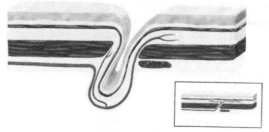

Fig. 5. Angioarchitecture of the blood supply of a diverticulum. A relatively large artery courses over the dome of the diverticulum and goes to the neck. Bleeding occurs along the course of this artery. In one study about three-fourths of bleeding occurred at the dome and only one-fourth was at the neck. (*From* Simpson PW, Nguyen MH, Lim JK, et al. Use of endoclips in the treatment of massive colonic diverticular bleeding. Gastrointest Endosc 2004;59:434; with permission.)

Treatment

The endoscopic treatment of a bleeding diverticulum is performed when stigmata of recent bleeding is found on colonoscopy. When an actively bleeding lesion was found, 67% of patients would rebleed.[14] When an adherent clot was found despite washing, 43% of patients would rebleed. Endoscopic band ligation, endoscopic clamping using the over-the-scope clip (OTSC), bipolar electrocoagulation, epinephrine injection, and endoscopic through-the-scope clipping (whether directly or from within a long cap) are some of the available techniques.

Note that colonic diverticula lack the muscular layer; therefore, bipolar electro-coagulation therapy is typically not used because of the risk of perforation.

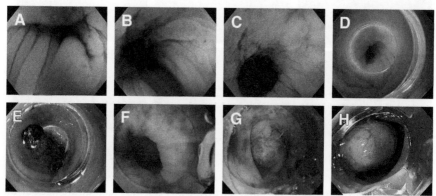

Fig. 6. Use of a long cap to invert a small-mouthed diverticulum. (*A*) The short distal attachment cap was used to investigate the many diverticula. Each diverticulum was washed with water jet while simultaneously using half-suction. (*B*) A large fresh clot was found. (*C*) The diverticulum had erosions on its neck but could not be inverted because the cap was too short. A clip was placed next to the diverticulum to mark the area and the endoscope was removed. (*D*) The endoscope was reinserted with a longer cap. (*E*) The clot was able to be suctioned out from the diverticulum. (*F*) The endoscope was equipped with a clamp device. (*G*) The erosion at the base of the dome was exposed. (*H*) After clamping.

Epinephrine injection monotherapy has a high risk of rebleeding (20%).[19] The choice of whether to use band ligation or clipping relies on availability, as well as device-use comfort and the size of the bleeding diverticula. A recent meta-analysis comparing the different endoscopic hemostasis modalities showed that banding was more effective than clipping to avoid interventional radiology or surgery.[19]

Band ligation: The potential to use endoscopic band ligation to treat the bleeding diverticulum is attractive[20] because most gastroenterologists are familiar with this technique and a large number of studies are now available to provide data on its safety and efficacy (**Fig. 7**).[19] Shimamura and colleagues[16] have shown that band ligation of bleeding diverticula can be performed by both expert and nonexpert (trainee) endoscopists with similar safety, efficacy (100%) and procedure time.

To perform band ligation, following identification of the bleeding diverticula and marking its location with an endoscopic clip, the endoscope is pulled out. Typically, the pediatric colonoscope is used to treat right-sided diverticula while the therapeutic upper endoscope is used for the left colon. The banding accessory is then attached. The bleeding diverticulum is reidentified and standard band ligation is performed. In a bleeding case, reinsertion of the colonoscope is often believed to be difficult. However, reinsertion is actually simpler because the colon has been straightened. The use of metal clips at the location allows for rapid reidentification of the bleeding diverticulum. Should bleeding become uncontrollable or recur, an abdominal radiograph that exposes the metal clip can provide the radiologist or surgeon with a precise location of the bleeding diverticulum.

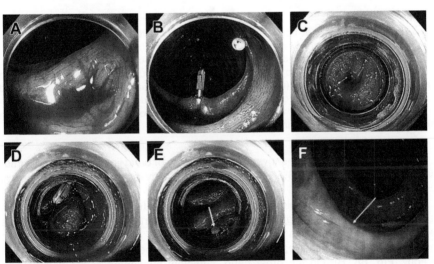

Fig. 7. Endoscopic band ligation of a bleeding colonic diverticulum. (*A*) Active bleeding was observed from a diverticulum in the ascending colon. (*B*) Marking clips were deployed at both sides of the diverticulum with stigmata of recent hemorrhage for easy identification on reinsertion of the colonoscope. (*C*) A band ligation device was attached to the tip of the colonoscope, the scope was reinserted, and the marked diverticulum was located. (*D*) The diverticulum was suctioned and 1 band was released. (*E*) A vessel was observed on the banded diverticulum (*arrow*). Bleeding stopped completely. (*F*) Typical appearance of a well-healed scar (*arrow*) weeks after band ligation.

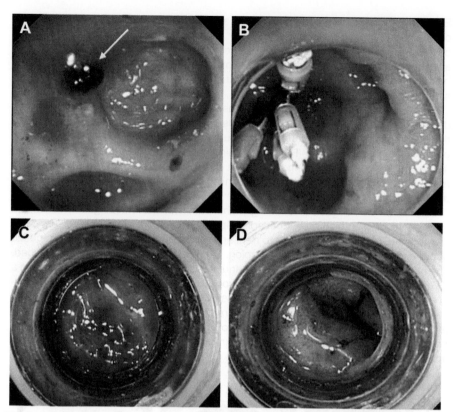

Fig. 8. Band ligation cannot be performed in all cases of diverticular bleeding. (*A*) A non-bleeding visible vessel (*arrow*) was seen in the dome of a giant diverticulum with a large orifice. Band ligation would not have worked in this case because the diverticulum was too large to be suctioned into the banding device. (*B*) Thus, direct endoscopic clipping was performed on the vessel. (*C*) In another case, band ligation could not be performed because the diverticulum was too small and its small orifice did not allow the diverticulum to be inverted. (*D*) Therefore, although less than ideal, the bleeding was treated using diluted epinephrine solution mixed with India ink.

In a pooled analysis, it was shown that the efficacy of band ligation to treat diverticular bleeding is up to 99% (95% CI 95%–100%) and early recurrent bleeding to be 9% (95% CI 4%–15%).[19]

In cases in which the bleeding diverticulum has too large or too small an orifice, band ligation cannot be performed. The diameter of the diverticula is required to be smaller than that of the band ligation device. In cases in which the diverticulum is massive, endoscopic clips can be deployed on the vessel directly (**Fig. 8**A, B). On the other hand, sufficient suctioning of the diverticulum is needed to complete band ligation. Because of this, it can be difficult to obtain sufficient suctioning of the diverticulum with an orifice that is too small. Other endoscopic treatments, such as epinephrine injection, are required for these lesions (**Fig. 8**C, D).

Ikeya and colleagues[21] reported that risk factors for early rebleeding after band ligation include younger age, active bleeding at the time of colonoscopy, and left-sided diverticula.

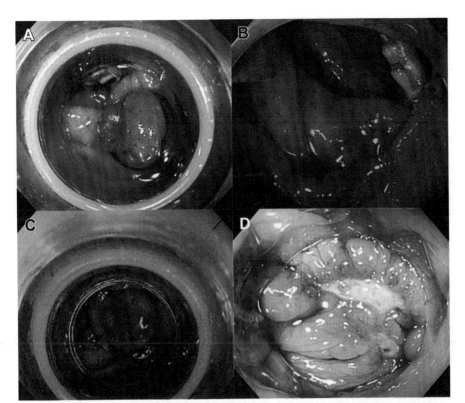

Fig. 9. Rebleeding after band ligation. (*A*) Band ligation was performed for actively bleeding diverticulum. The band was deployed without adequate suctioning of the diverticulum and a complete eversion of the diverticulum was not achieved. (*B*) Rebleeding occurred 1 day after band ligation. Repeat colonoscopy showed the band was not present. (*C*) Band ligation was repeated, this time after sufficient suctioning and eversion of the diverticulum. (*D*) In another case, recurrent bleeding occurred 10 days after band ligation. Repeat colonoscopy demonstrated an ulcer at the prior banding site. No additional treatment was performed because the ulcer was clean based. (*Courtesy of* Yasutoshi Shiratori, MD, Department of Gastroenterology, St. Luke's International Hospital, Tokyo, Japan; with permission.)

Typically, when bleeding occurs after band ligation, a repeat colonoscopy is performed to evaluate the cause. For early dislodgement of the band, repeat ligation is performed (**Fig. 9**A–C). However, repeat band ligation can be performed only for the diverticulum in which the band dislodges at an early phase and ulceration does not occur at the banded site. When there is ulcer formation at the site, repeat band ligation is not typically performed (**Fig. 9**D). Instead, clipping is done when there is a visible vessel within the ulcer at the banded site. When the banded site appears yellowish or blackish, we watch and wait. It should be noted that necrotic tissue is not removed after band ligation in the rebleeding cases because the banded tissue may contain the underlying muscularis propria and snaring has a theoretical risk of perforation.

Band ligation of the bleeding diverticulum had been reported to cause a delayed perforation in a patient who was on chronic steroid therapy and aspirin[22] and to lead to uncomplicated diverticulitis in another.[23] Thus, ligation may not be indicated when wound healing is inhibited.

There are some limitations to using the band ligation device to treat bleeding diverticula. In the United States, most units supply the upper band ligation kits, in which case the trigger cord is not long enough for a colonoscope. Thus, treatment of a bleeding right-sided diverticula may be more difficult to perform. Endoscopic views become limited after the band has been attached. To mitigate the limited views, a preference is given to the clear-view type of bander, and to deploy or get rid of four bands before insertion of the endoscope.

Clipping: At least four different techniques of clipping have been described, including (1) direct clipping onto the bleeding diverticular vessel, (2) clipping along the neck when stigmata is within the dome, (3) clipping the mouth of the diverticulum shut when the stigmata is seen or is presumed to be within the dome, and (4) clipping from within the cap (used to invert the diverticula to expose the stigmata). Rebleeding, however, has been reported to be more common when clipping was not directed to clip the bleeding stigmata.

Direct clipping can be performed without withdrawal and reinsertion of the colonoscope. The technique is especially useful when the bleeding stigmata are at the neck. When the stigmata are at the dome, direct clipping is more difficult and care must be taken so that the clip does not inadvertently puncture the dome.

Indirect placement of endoscopic clips is sometimes performed around the neck or in a zipper fashion due to the difficulty of direct placement of the clips at the source in the dome (**Fig. 10**). However, indirect placement is ineffective to occlude the ruptured vasa recta at the diverticulum and sometimes cannot control bleeding, especially when the diverticulum is in the ascending colon.[24] Because indirect clipping has the highest risk of rebleeding, the authors prefer direct placement of endoscopic clips.

Clipping from within a cap: The cap can be extremely useful in such cases because the dome is inverted into it (see **Fig. 3**). Clipping can be precisely done in these cases. However, the required cap is the longer length type, similar to the cap used for band ligation.

Clamping: The safety and efficacy of OTSC to treat diverticular bleeding have been described.[25–28] The OTSC offers several advantages over the banding or through-the-scope clipping methods, including (1) OTSC is made for the colonoscope

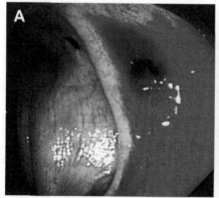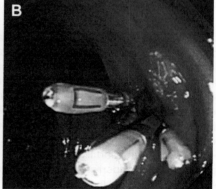

Fig. 10. Indirect endoscopic clipping method of a bleeding colonic diverticulum. The entire diverticulum was clipped shut. (*A*) Active bleeding with a clot was observed from a diverticulum in the ascending colon. (*B*) The diverticulum was closed in a zipper fashion with four clips and bleeding stopped.

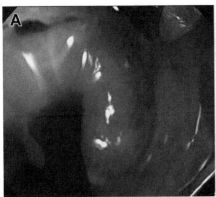 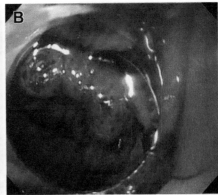

Fig. 11. Use of over-the-scope clip for active bleeding from diverticular dome. (*A*) Active bleeding was seen from the dome area of a small mouthed diverticulum. (*B*) An OTSC was used. The diverticulum was everted into the cap, and then the clamp was deployed to ligate the diverticulum and the bleeding stopped.

so it fits tightly onto the scope and the trip cord is of the appropriate length; (2) viewing is better; and (3) placement is more secure, if not permanent (**Fig. 11**).

Long-term outcomes

Kaltenbach and colleagues[3] reported long-term outcomes using endoscopic clipping techniques. Recurrent bleeding occurred beyond 30 days in about 24% of patients during 35 plus or minus 18 months of follow-up.[3] Nakano and colleagues[29] have reported the cumulative rebleeding rates as high as 41% at 36 months after band ligation and that the recurrence appeared to originate from other diverticula. These data suggest that, in some patients, diverticular bleeding is a recurrent disease and current endoscopic treatment is useful as an emergency measure but does not always address the long-term bleeding recurrence.[7]

Postpolypectomy bleeding

Postpolypectomy bleeding typically presents as self-limited hematochezia within the first 36 hours following a polypectomy. Pooled prevalence data from 21 studies, including close to 2 million colonoscopies performed over the period of 2001 to 2012, show a postpolypectomy bleeding rate of 9.8 per 1000 (95% CI 7.7–12.1).[30] Significant risk factors for postpolypectomy bleeding include polyp size greater than 10 mm, pedunculated polyps with thick stalks, sessile lateral spreading polyps, right-sided colonic lesions, use of anticoagulants, and patient comorbidities such as cardiovascular or chronic renal disease. Colonoscopy in such patients may show a postpolypectomy ulcer site with active bleeding, clot, or red spot. The postpolypectomy site is clipped closed, although, more recently, clamping has also been used (**Fig. 12**). The authors also clip bleeding that occurs after endoscopic submucosal dissection (**Fig. 13**).

The key to postpolypectomy bleeding is prevention. Large polyps (>20 mm) or pedunculated polyps with a thick stalk have a higher bleeding risk. Prophylactic ligation of the blood vessel of the large stalk has been shown to reduce immediate and/or delayed bleeding. One prophylactic method is the endoloop technique.[31] An endoloop is a detachable nylon loop that can be applied to the base of polyp stalk to strangulate the feeding vessel of the polyp. Other endoscopists have reported clipping of the stalk before polypectomy, although completely clipping across a large stalk may be

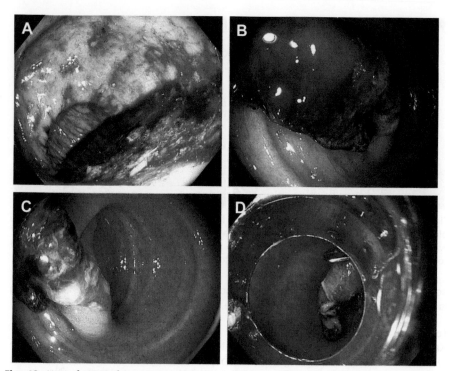

Fig. 12. Use of OTSC for primary hemostasis of postpolypectomy bleeding. (*A*) Bloody effluent was seen throughout the colon despite rapid bowel purge, suggestive of ongoing active bleeding. (*B*) Postpolypectomy site of a 1.5 cm pedunculated polyp that was hot snared the day before can be seen with a large clot and active bleeding. (*C*) Epinephrine was injected to cold snare the clot (*D*) An OTSC was placed at the stalk base to ligate the large feeding vessel.

challenging.[32] A randomized trial among 195 subjects with pedunculated polyps with a minimum stalk diameter of 5 mm showed a similar bleeding rate following prophylaxis with placement of an endoloop (5.7%) or clips (5.1%).[33] Readers are directed to the review by two of the current authors, Kaltenbach and Soetikno,[2] on how to perform resection of large polyps and how to prevent the bleeding complications.

Arteriovenous malformation

AVM can present with acute severe LGIB, yet it typically presents as occult bleeding. Slightly more than 25% of patients with colonic AVM have more than one lesion. APC has been the most frequently used treatment modality. Note the importance of bowel preparation in patients undergoing APC anywhere in the colon and rectum because of the risk of methane gas explosion. Typical settings of APC are 30 W and 1.2 L per minute gas flow rate. Because the colon is thinnest in the right colon, submucosal saline injection has been used to provide cushioning before performing APC on AVMs greater than 10 mm. The efficacy of APC has been reported to be higher than 85%.

The authors, and others, use clipping to treat the bleeding colonic AVM because clipping does not cause tissue injury. Clipping, however, requires precision, thus multiple clips are placed in a zipper-like configuration to treat colonic AVM (**Fig. 14**).

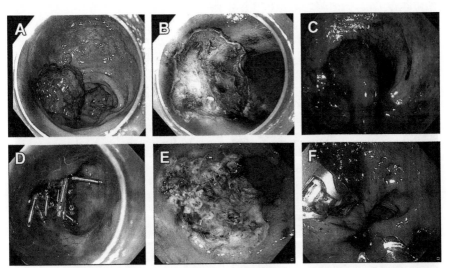

Fig. 13. Bleeding after endoscopic submucosal dissection (ESD) in a patient on anticoagulation. (*A*) A large recurrent rectal adenoma was seen in the proximal rectum. (*B*) Endoscopic submucosal dissection was performed because the lesion was not lifting after submucosal injection. (*C*) The patient presented five days later with acute LGIB. After rapid bowel purge, a sigmoidoscopy was performed. A large adherent blood clot was found at the ESD site. (*D*) The bleeding was treated with diluted epinephrine injection and multiple endoscopic clips were placed. (*E*) Rebreeding occurred four days later and sigmoidoscopy was repeated. Most of the clips had fallen off (likely due to scarring from multiple prior resections) but there were two remaining clips that were removed with rat tooth forceps to expose the defect fully. (*F*) A visible vessel was identified. The bleeding was treated successfully with endoscopic suturing.

Miscellaneous

Dieulafoy bleeding
Although rare, Dieulafoy bleeding may be profuse and intermittent. As such, treatment to the Dieulafoy artery is preferred with either banding[34] or (preferably) clamping using the OTSC.[4]

Hemorrhoidal bleeding
Hemorrhoidal bleeding can rarely be severe. Band ligation is the preferred technique. Soetikno and colleagues[4] recently reported the use of OTSC to treat bleeding posthemorrhoidectomy. Precision is required in banding or clamping in the transition zone of anal canal to avoid banding or clamping the squamous mucosa.

Ischemia, inflammatory bowel disease, and neoplastic bleeding
Colonoscopy can be helpful in the diagnosis of the potential bleeding sources of ischemia, inflammatory bowel disease, and neoplastic bleeding (see **Fig. 12**). Bleeding, however, is typically diffuse and self-limited. Pinpoint bleeding for colorectal cancer is usually amenable to APC or even clipping.

Use of interventional radiology and surgery
There are times when LGIB is not amenable to endoscopic therapy. Emphasis on a multidisciplinary team approach with close collaboration between the gastroenterologist, radiologist, surgeon, and internist is the recommended approach to acute severe lower GI bleed.

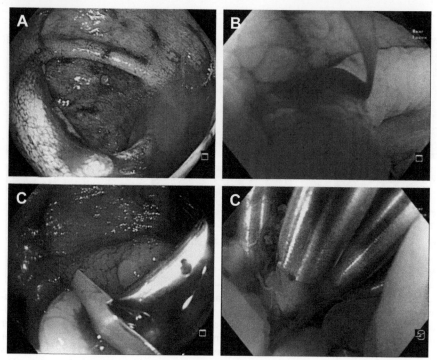

Fig. 14. Endoscopic direct clipping for primary hemostasis of AVM bleeding in a patient with von Willebrand disease. (*A*) A pool of fresh blood with active bleeding was seen in the cecum following rapid bowel purge. (*B*) With water irrigation, the focal bleeding source, which was an AVM, was identified. (*C*) Direct clipping at the site. (*D*) Multiple clips were applied for complete hemostasis.

CONCLUSION

When the authors first presented the use of endoclips in the treatment of massive diverticular bleeding in the Video Forum during Digestive Disease Week in the early 2000s, the moderator of the session asked if they were lucky or if they good. The question went unanswered. Thinking back, they had turned their heads into the unknown and were successful primarily because they were driven by the fear of the use of an old treatment modality. The patient, a 77-year-old quadriplegic man who had received 12 units of packed red blood cells for severe lower gastrointestinal bleeding, was being wheeled to the operating room for a subtotal colectomy. They embraced the new technique, the endoclips, which was not widely used at that time, to stop the bleeding. The authors asked the surgeons to give them a chance and placed two clips (Case 1).[1] The patient never had recurrent bleeding.

Since that time, significant progress has been made in the techniques to diagnose and to treat severe LGIB. These techniques can be applied in the appropriate settings. However, few robust studies have been performed to date to confirm its safety and efficacy beyond the expert centers. Further data are needed to fully recommend the use of colonoscopy in the urgent or emergent setting. The foundations, which we have described in this article, are available for these studies to be completed.

REFERENCES

1. Simpson PW, Nguyen MH, Lim JK, et al. Use of endoclips in the treatment of massive colonic diverticular bleeding. Gastrointest Endosc 2004;59(3):433–7.

2. Kaltenbach T, Soetikno R. Endoscopic resection of large colon polyps. Gastrointest Endosc Clin N Am 2013;23(1):137–52.
3. Kaltenbach T, Watson R, Shah J, et al. Colonoscopy with clipping is useful in the diagnosis and treatment of diverticular bleeding. Clin Gastroenterol Hepatol 2012;10(2):131–7.
4. Soetikno R, Asokkumar R, Sim D, et al. Use of the over-the-scope clip to treat massive bleeding at the transitional zone of the anal canal: a case series. Gastrointest Endosc 2016;84(1):168–72.
5. Soetikno R, Kaltenbach T, Friedland S. Endoscopic appearance of bleeding diverticula and treatment with endoscopic clipping. 2006.
6. Soetikno R, Kaltenbach T, Kelsey P, et al. Endoscopic interpretation and therapy to severe lower gastrointestinal bleeding, 2008.
7. Soetikno R, Wu C, Kaltenbach T. Is there an optimal technique to treat the bleeding diverticulum? Is diverticular bleeding a recurrent disease? Endosc Int Open 2015;3(5):E534–5.
8. Barkun AN, Martel M. The role of early colonoscopy in acute lower GI bleeding: summarizing conflicting data in the presence of society recommendations. Gastrointest Endosc 2017;86(1):118–9.
9. Sanchez A. Middle gastrointestinal bleeding. In: Tony C. K. Tham, JSAC, Roy M. Soetikno, editors. Gastrointestinal emergencies. 3rd edition. p. 230–238.
10. Bardou M, Benhaberou-Brun D, Le Ray I, et al. Diagnosis and management of nonvariceal upper gastrointestinal bleeding. Nat Rev Gastroenterol Hepatol 2012;9(2):97–104.
11. Blatchford O, Murray WR, Blatchford M. A risk score to predict need for treatment for upper-gastrointestinal haemorrhage. Lancet 2000;356(9238):1318–21.
12. Strate LL, Saltzman JR, Ookubo R, et al. Validation of a clinical prediction rule for severe acute lower intestinal bleeding. Am J Gastroenterol 2005;100(8):1821–7.
13. Strate LL, Gralnek IM. ACG clinical guideline: management of patients with acute lower gastrointestinal bleeding. Am J Gastroenterol 2016;111(4):459–74.
14. Jensen DM, Machicado GA, Jutabha R, et al. Urgent colonoscopy for the diagnosis and treatment of severe diverticular hemorrhage. N Engl J Med 2000; 342(2):78–82.
15. Jensen DM, Machicado GA. Diagnosis and treatment of severe hematochezia. The role of urgent colonoscopy after purge. Gastroenterology 1988;95(6): 1569–74.
16. Shimamura Y, Ishii N, Omata F, et al. Endoscopic band ligation for colonic diverticular bleeding: possibility of standardization. Endosc Int open 2016;4(2):E233–7.
17. Ueno S, Nakase H, Kasahara K, et al. Clinical features of Japanese patients with colonic angiodysplasia. J Gastroenterol Hepatol 2008;23(8 Pt 2):e363–6.
18. Ishii N, Itoh T, Uemura M, et al. Endoscopic band ligation with a water-jet scope for the treatment of colonic diverticular hemorrhage. Dig Endosc 2010;22(3):232–5.
19. Ishii N, Omata F, Nagata N, et al. Effectiveness of endoscopic treatments for colonic diverticular bleeding. Gastrointest Endosc 2018;87(1):58–66.
20. Farrell JJ, Graeme-Cook F, Kelsey PB. Treatment of bleeding colonic diverticula by endoscopic band ligation: an in-vivo and ex-vivo pilot study. Endoscopy 2003;35(10):823–9.
21. Ikeya T, Ishii N, Nakano K, et al. Risk factors for early rebleeding after endoscopic band ligation for colonic diverticular hemorrhage. Endosc Int open 2015;3(5): E523–8.
22. Takahashi S, Inaba T, Tanaka N. Delayed perforation after endoscopic band ligation for treatment of colonic diverticular bleeding. Dig Endosc 2016;28(4):484.

23. Ishii N, Fujita Y. Colonic diverticulitis after endoscopic band ligation performed for colonic diverticular hemorrhage. ACG Case Rep J 2015;2(4):218–20.

24. Ishii N, Hirata N, Omata F, et al. Location in the ascending colon is a predictor of refractory colonic diverticular hemorrhage after endoscopic clipping. Gastrointest Endosc 2012;76(6):1175–81.

25. Kassab I, Dressner R, Gorcey S. Over-the-scope clip for control of a recurrent diverticular bleed. ACG case Rep J 2015;3(1):5–6.

26. Probst A, Braun G, Goelder S, et al. Endoscopic treatment of colonic diverticular bleeding using an over-the-scope clip. Endoscopy 2016;48(Suppl 1):E160.

27. Wedi E, von Renteln D, Jung C, et al. Treatment of acute colonic diverticular bleeding in high risk patients, using an over-the-scope clip: a case series. Endoscopy 2016;48(S 01):E383–5.

28. Kolb JM, Kaltenbach T, Soetikno RM. 935 endoscopic clipping technique using the over the scope clip to treat diverticular bleeding. Gastrointest Endosc 2016; 83(5):AB188–AB89.

29. Nakano K, Ishii N, Ikeya T, et al. Comparison of long-term outcomes between endoscopic band ligation and endoscopic clipping for colonic diverticular hemorrhage. Endosc Int Open 2015;03(05):E529–33.

30. Reumkens A, Rondagh EJ, Bakker CM, et al. Post-colonoscopy complications: a systematic review, time trends, and meta-analysis of population-based studies. Am J Gastroenterol 2016;111(8):1092–101.

31. Iishi H, Tatsuta M, Narahara H, et al. Endoscopic resection of large pedunculated colorectal polyps using a detachable snare. Gastrointest Endosc 1996;44(5): 594–7.

32. Kouklakis G, Mpoumponaris A, Gatopoulou A, et al. Endoscopic resection of large pedunculated colonic polyps and risk of postpolypectomy bleeding with adrenaline injection versus endoloop and hemoclip: a prospective, randomized study. Surg Endosc 2009;23(12):2732–7.

33. Ji JS, Lee SW, Kim TH, et al. Comparison of prophylactic clip and endoloop application for the prevention of postpolypectomy bleeding in pedunculated colonic polyps: a prospective, randomized, multicenter study. Endoscopy 2014;46(7): 598–604.

34. Vandervoort J, Montes H, Soetikno RM, et al. Use of endoscopic band ligation in the treatment of ongoing rectal bleeding. Gastrointest Endosc 1999;49(3 Pt 1): 392–4.

Prevention of Recurrent Lower Gastrointestinal Hemorrhage

Shivani Gupta, MD*, David A. Greenwald, MD

KEYWORDS

- Lower GI bleeding • Prevention of recurrent LGIB • Diverticular bleeding
- Angioectasia • Chronic hemorrhagic radiation proctopathy
- Postpolypectomy bleeding • Endoscopic therapy

KEY POINTS

- The majority of diverticular bleeding self-resolves, but the risk of recurrent hemorrhage remains high. Diverticula with high-risk stigmata (active bleeding, nonbleeding visible vessel, or adherent clot) are particularly prone to rebleeding and should be endoscopically treated.
- Argon plasma coagulation (APC) is a proved and safe modality for the treatment of angioectasia, but rebleed rates remain high.
- Chronic hemorrhagic radiation proctopathy is amenable to endoscopic therapy, preferably APC. Given the potential associated morbidity, however, endoscopic therapy should be used judiciously.
- The practice of placing clips after endoscopic mucosal resection (EMR) of polyps to avoid delayed bleeding remains contentious. Yet, there may be utility in clipping, particularly for large lesions or for individuals requiring anticoagulation after polypectomy.
- Nonsteroidal anti-inflammatory drugs (NSAIDs) should be discontinued, if possible, especially in cases of lower gastrointestinal bleeding (LGIB) due to diverticulosis and angioectasia, due to the high rebleed risk. Aspirin should be continued if medically indicated. The management of other antiplatelet agents or anticoagulants must be tailored to the patient and often requires a multidisciplinary approach.

INTRODUCTION

Lower gastrointestinal bleeding (LGIB) encompasses all bleeds involving the colon extending from the ileocecal valve to the anus.[1] Overt LGIB most commonly manifests as hematochezia but may also present as melena in proximal colonic bleeds.[2] The major modality for diagnosing the etiology of LGIB is colonoscopy, which allows for direct

Disclosure Statement: None.
Division of Gastroenterology, Icahn School of Medicine at Mount Sinai, Mount Sinai Hospital, One Gustave L. Levy Place, Box 1069, New York, NY 10029-6574, USA
* Corresponding author.
E-mail address: shivani.gupta@mountsinai.org

visualization of the colonic mucosa and the ability to perform immediate therapeutic maneuvers to achieve hemostasis.[2] Alternatively, imaging studies, including CT angiography (CTA) with catheter-directed embolization, may be used, particularly in situations where there are barriers to endoscopic evaluation.[2] These barriers include significant comorbidities, clinical instability in which patients are unable to undergo sufficient bowel preparation,[2] patient or family preference, and ongoing obscure bleeding despite endoscopic evaluation.[3]

Radiologic studies, such as tagged red blood cell radionuclide scans are relatively sensitive for the presence of gastrointestinal (GI) bleeding, with the ability to identify bleeding that is occurring at rates as low as 0.1 mL/min.[1] In addition, this study may be performed several times over the course of a day if there is difficulty identifying the etiology of an intermittent bleed.[1] Radionuclide scans, however, are a blunt diagnostic tool and can only suggest the general region of a bleed, which limits its utility.[1]

Alternatively, mesenteric angiography may detect bleeding at rates greater than 0.5 mL/min and allows for therapeutic intervention with catheter-guided embolization or injection of vasoactive substances.[1] The major downsides are that there is a non-negligible incidence of colonic infarction with therapy[1] **(Fig. 1)** as well as risk of contrast-induced nephropathy.[4]

REBLEED RISK

LGIB is a frequent condition, resulting in the hospitalization of 21 per 100,000 individuals each year,[4] and carries a significant risk of recurrence.[3] Predisposing determinants of recurrent LGIB include the modality used to achieve primary hemostasis[5]; the use of antiplatelet agents, nonsteroidal anti-inflammatory drugs (NSAIDs), and anticoagulants[5]; the presence of end-stage renal disease or cirrhosis[5]; and the etiology of the initial bleed.[2] It is not well established what the proportionate impact of these individual characteristics is on the incidence of recurrent bleeding.[5]

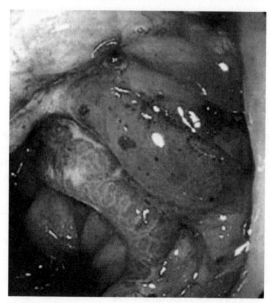

Fig. 1. Evidence of colonic ischemia after transcatheter glue embolization of the left colic artery for persistent diverticular bleeding.

In 1 retrospective study between 1985 and 2002 involving 171 patients with severe acute LGIB[a] (specified in this study as hematochezia with decline in hematocrit of 10 or more points or receipt of a minimum transfusion of 3 units packed red blood cells) presenting to a tertiary medical facility, more than half of individuals had experienced prior hematochezia.[3] Of the cases in which the bleeding source was identified, diverticulosis was the most common, followed by anorectal disease and angiodysplasia.[3] Notably, 15% of subjects were on antiplatelet medications and 9% on anticoagulants at the time of study inclusion.[3] Over the course of a mean follow-up of 11 years, approximately one-third of participants (n = 52) had recurrent LGIB, of which the predominant sources in identified cases were diverticulosis (n = 17), angiodysplasia (n = 9), and rectal varicose veins (n = 4).[3]

DISEASE-SPECIFIC RISK AND PREVENTION
Diverticulosis

Diverticulosis is the most frequent etiology of hemorrhage of the lower GI tract, constituting 30% to 65% of cases.[4] Diverticular bleeding typically is painless, occurs in 3% to 5% of individuals with diverticulosis, and tends to affect middle-aged to elderly patients (50–70 years).[1] Most diverticular bleeding episodes, approximately 75%, resolve without intervention.[1] The recurrence rate, however, is 15% to 20% after the first diverticular bleed and increases to 25% to 50% after the second occurrence.[1] In particular, visualization of active hemorrhage during endoscopy or the presence of an adherent clot or a nonbleeding visible vessel, predisposes to recurrent hemorrhage if no intervention is performed.[2] Identification of these high-risk endoscopic features is an indication for endoscopic treatment.[2]

Yet, as is well known by endoscopists, the localization of the culprit diverticulum is onerous and typically elusive, successfully occurring in only 6% to 42% of patients.[6] Exacerbating conditions include the length of the colon, the on-off nature of the hemorrhage, the burden of diverticular disease, and the presence of obscuring fecal material or blood.[6] To improve detection of these high-risk features, complete bowel preparation, short time to colonoscopic evaluation (within 24 hours of patient presentation), and use of a cap on the tip of the colonoscope should be considered.[6]

ENDOSCOPIC PREVENTION OF RECURRENT DIVERTICULAR BLEEDS

Endoscopic treatment modalities for diverticular bleeding include application of thermal coagulation or mechanical clip placement, either alone or in conjunction with mucosal epinephrine injection, or band ligation.[2] Endoscopic clipping may be of particular value due to a lower risk of perforation in the delicate colon as opposed to contact thermal coagulation.[2] Clips may be deployed specifically over the high-risk endoscopic stigmata or placed in such a manner as to fully seal off the culprit diverticulum.[2] Regardless of the primary management technique used, it is recommended that the index diverticulum be marked with either an India ink tattoo or an endoscopic clip to help identify the lesion in the event of recurrent hemorrhage.[2]

In a 2010 report on the endoscopic management of diverticular hemorrhage, Strate and Naumann[4] identified 137 patients, of whom the largest number had undergone

---

[a] Included 12 small bowel bleeds.

clip placement (n = 71). Cessation of bleeding with endoscopic therapeutic techniques was achieved in 92% of subjects (100% of individuals undergoing clip placement).[4] The overall rate of early (≤30 days)[7] recurrent hemorrhage was 8%[4]; late hemorrhage occurred in 12%.[4] The placement of clips was associated with no early recurrent hemorrhage but a 17% incidence of late recurrent bleed.[4] Another study (n = 87), however, demonstrated an early recurrent hemorrhage rate of 34% with clip placement.[8]

In the contact thermal coagulation cohort (n = 17 subjects), the early and late recurrent hemorrhage rates were 12% and 0%, respectively.[4] In the epinephrine monotherapy group (n = 20), the incidence of early and late recurrent hemorrhage rates were 15% and 5%, respectively.[4] As with upper GI bleeding pathology, epinephrine injection by itself is not viewed as a definitive therapy and has a high chance of early recurrent hemorrhage.[6]

Finally, dual therapy with dilute epinephrine injection followed by thermal coagulation did not seem to diminish early or late rebleeding rates (n = 25 subjects, 24% and 16%, respectively)[4] compared with either modality alone.[2] Instead, epinephrine injection may have a role in enhancing success of endoscopic clipping by assisting in constricting bleeding vessels and possibly raising the contents of the diverticulum into view to allow for targeted clipping.[2]

A novel approach to managing diverticular bleeding is endoscopic band ligation (EBL). A retrospective investigation in a Tokyo hospital, involving 29 subjects and 31 colonic diverticula with high-risk features (active bleeding, nonbleeding visible vessel, or adherent clot), examined treatment efficacy of EBL.[7] EBL was performed in 87% of the diverticula, excluding 4 cases in which the large size of either the dome or opening of the diverticulum precluded band deployment.[7] Clip placement or epinephrine administration was then used instead.[7]

In this study, the rate of early recurrent hemorrhage for EBL was 11%.[7] In 1 of these relapses, failure to initially band the entire diverticulum resulted in a repeat bleed on post-treatment day one, which was rectified with recurrent banding.[7] Over a mean of 11 months post-treatment, there was only 1 episode of late recurrent hemorrhage.[7] Notably, 11 subjects underwent repeat colonoscopy after 6 months or 1 year, and there was demonstrated scarring at the site of the prior diverticulum in 7 of these individuals.[7] In the remaining 4, the position of the formerly banded diverticulum was unable to be located.[7] Thus, the investigators hypothesized that late recurrent hemorrhage was possibly averted due to post-treatment eradication of the involved diverticulum.[7]

One concerning complication of EBL is the possibility of strangulating full-thickness colon, particularly in the treatment of proximal (right colon) diverticula.[2] This risk seems minimal, however, with no reported instances of perforation.[6]

Due to small sample sizes in most trials and a deficit of prospective head to head trials, it is difficult to discern the superiority of 1 endoscopic treatment over another for both primary hemostasis and prophylaxis against rebleeding in diverticular hemorrhage. Moreover, it is questionable whether endoscopic interventions are truly effective in preventing repeat lower gastrointestinal (LGI) hemorrhage as a different diverticulum may subsequently bleed.[2] The best evidence, however, seems to exist for the use of endoscopic clipping in the treatment of diverticular hemorrhage, particularly given the lower chance of perforation relative to contact thermal coagulation.[2] Data are also emerging to support EBL as a possible viable option, although this requires the appropriate anatomic compatibility of the bleeding diverticulum.

One investigation demonstrates at least indirect evidence that treatment of the culprit diverticulum prevents rebleeding from that same diverticulum. In a retrospective study spanning close to 20 years, 37 of 78 subjects with diverticular bleeding (excluding 17 subjects who proceeded to colectomy) experienced rebleeding after a median of 8.1 months[9]; 84% of these individuals bled from the same location, 5% from another location, and 11% from an unknown point in the colon.[9] The majority of these subjects (n = 63) had not undergone therapeutic intervention to achieve primary hemostasis because these bleeds had self-resolved.[9] Only 10 individuals had endoscopic techniques used to achieve hemostasis during the first episode of LGIB, and 7 experienced repeat hemorrhage.[9]

Angioectasia

Angioectasia, also referred to as angiodysplasias and arteriovenous malformations,[10] are identified in 3% to 6% of individuals in whom colonoscopy is performed[1] and constitute 7% of cases of overt colonic hemorrhage.[11] These lesions are most often seen in the ascending colon and cecum.[1] Angioectasia incidence increases with age, but the vast majority (approximately 90%) of individuals do not manifest any signs of bleeding, including occult blood loss.[1] Of those who do bleed, most resolve without intervention,[12] but there is a high chance of recurrent hemorrhage.[13]

Often, individuals respond to iron supplementation alone.[1] If pursued, endoscopic ablative techniques, such as argon plasma coagulation (APC), often are successful in achieving hemostasis and obliterating lesions[1,13] (**Fig. 2**). But, rebleeding approaches 50%.[13] The management of angioectasia poses difficulty because several of these vascular malformations may be present concurrently[10] and may subsequently develop in new locations.[2]

MEDICAL THERAPY

Overall, high-quality data are lacking to support routine use of medical therapy, including thalidomide, hormonal therapy, and octreotide, in the setting of angioectasia,[11] particularly given the increased incidence of adverse events.[2] In particularly difficult endoscopic situations, however, such as high angioectasia burden or inability to achieve hemostasis due to angioectasia location within the GI tract, medical therapy with the aforementioned agents may be considered.[11,14]

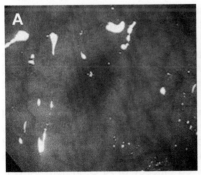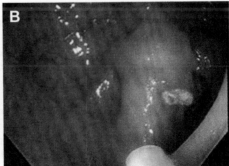

Fig. 2. (A) Sigmoid angioectasia detected as part of the diagnostic work-up for iron deficiency anemia. No active bleeding seen at the time of the examination. (B) Sigmoid angioectasia post-APC.

ENDOSCOPIC PREVENTION OF RECURRENT OCCULT OR OVERT BLEEDING

Endoscopic treatment is the preferred therapy for symptomatic angioectasia[13] and is warranted for both overt or occult bleeding,[2,13] which may manifest as iron deficiency anemia.[13] Experts advise against attempting endoscopic eradication of asymptomatic lesions, because such findings are associated with a relatively low incidence of bleeding.[10,12,13] In 1 retrospective cohort study, of 15 subjects with incidentally identified angioectasia on colonoscopy, none had LGIB over a mean 2-year period.[15]

For endoscopic treatment of angioectasia, APC is often the preferred modality due to its favorable risk profile.[2,14] With APC, primary hemostasis is achieved in 85% of cases,[10] and there is a decreased need for repeat transfusions.[2] Other treatment options include contact thermal approaches, such as heater probe and monopolar thermal coagulation.[2] Heater probe use has been associated with proximal colonic perforations[13] but is generally equally efficacious as APC in achieving hemostasis.[10] The perforation rate using monopolar coagulation, which is much less frequently used, is 3%.[13] In contrast, APC is designed to deliver energy more superficially and thus is less prone to this complication.[13] Finally, mechanical clipping, possibly in conjunction with APC or contact thermal coagulation, has been used in the management of particularly large angioectasia as well as in individuals receiving antithrombotic therapy[10]; this technique may be considered in select cases.[10]

The risk of recurrent hemorrhage after endoscopic hemostasis in angioectasia is approximately 14% to 53% in the first 3 years and increases thereafter.[12] A systematic review published in 2014 was unable to conclude if any of the endoscopic interventions reduced recurrent hemorrhage versus conservative management.[11] Most of the available data are derived from retrospective investigations with few subjects,[11] thereby making the analysis problematic.

One such example is a small retrospective study involving 62 subjects who presented with overtly bleeding angioectasia from anywhere within the GI tract.[14] This investigation assessed rates of rebleeding between those undergoing exclusive conservative therapy (transfusions, iron supplementation, correction of coagulopathies, and so forth) versus conservative measures plus APC.[14] All angioectasia seen to be bleeding at the time of endoscopy were treated with APC.[14] Furthermore, the endoscopist had discretion as to whether to administer APC for nonbleeding angioectasia, contingent on frequency of prior bleeding, gravity of the current presentation, and other clinical factors.[14] APC was performed in 60% of analyzed subjects, although only approximately two-thirds of these individuals were acutely hemorrhaging at the time of endoscopic therapy.[14] Over an average 3-year period, 30% of individuals had a repeat hemorrhage, and the overwhelming majority were from the same location.[14] The rebleeding incidence was 21% for those treated with APC and 44% for individuals in the conservative treatment group ($P = .06$).[14] On multivariable analysis, multiple prior bleeds, over-anticoagulation based on prothrombin time, and more than 1 identified angioectasia on endoscopy were associated with a higher likelihood of repeat bleeding.[14] Use of APC was close to but did not meet statistical significance for decreasing repeat hemorrhage.[14]

The interpretation of these results is somewhat limited given the inclusion of bleeding proximal to the colon and the reliance on retrospective data,[14] which may lead to disparate treatment arms.[14] The groups seem to have been skewed so that those more likely to experience recurrent bleeding (ie, high-risk individuals) were treated with APC, thus diminishing the perceived efficacy of APC. In sum, APC is beneficial in limiting the need for transfusions[2] and may be successful in protecting against repeat hemorrhage, but further studies are required.

Radiation Proctopathy

The onset of chronic radiation proctopathy after radiation treatment ranges from 5% to 30%,[16,17] with many estimates favoring the higher end of the spectrum.[16] This complication occurs less frequently than previously, because administration of radiation for GI and genitourinary cancers has become more precise.[16,17] Several factors are correlated with the development of chronic radiation proctopathy. These include the amount of radiation given,[16,17] the quantity of total[16,17] and rectal tissue irradiated,[16] cancer stage,[16] other treatments received,[16] and the presence of comorbidities,[16,17] such as diabetes, vasculopathy, and inflammatory bowel disease.[17]

Radiation proctopathy may be divided into acute (occurring at the time of and for a maximum of 6 months after cessation of radiation) and chronic phases (either an extension of acute symptoms vs new onset after a minimum of 3 months),[16] the latter of which is the focus of this section. Symptoms of chronic radiation proctopathy include rectal discomfort, hematochezia, stricture formation, loss of sphincter control, and, infrequently, perforation or fistula formation.[16] The incidence of hemorrhage in chronic radiation proctopathy is 6% to 8%.[18] LGIB associated with radiation proctopathy may be delayed, sometimes occurring years after completion of radiation treatment.[1] Hematochezia, however, frequently ceases without intervention.[19]

Endoscopic characteristics of radiation proctopathy include pale mucosa, which easily bleeds, and the presence of telangiectasias[16,17] (**Fig. 3**). If biopsy specimens are deemed necessary, care should be taken when obtaining those mucosal samples because of the risk of fistula formation.[16,17] It is recommended that biopsies be taken from areas least exposed to prior radiation (ie, the posterior and lateral walls in those treated for prostate cancer).[16]

Medical Therapy

Medical therapy for chronic radiation proctopathy is associated with a favorable safety profile, so generally it is considered first-line treatment if conservative measures are unsuccessful.[17] Medications commonly used include oral or topical 5-aminosalicylic acid with or without topical or oral steroids, sucralfate enemas, oral metronidazole, short chain fatty acid enemas, vitamin A, formalin, and hyperbaric oxygen, all with varying efficacies.[16] The best evidence exists for the use of metronidazole, sucralfate enemas, and hyperbaric oxygen.[17] Sucralfate works by creating a physical barrier against potentially injurious substances and promoting vascular growth, thereby assisting in mucosal recovery.[17]

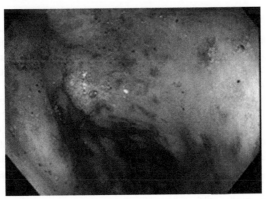

Fig. 3. Radiation proctopathy in an asymptomatic patient. No intervention pursued.

In 1 investigation by Kochhar and colleagues,[20] 26 subjects post-treatment of cervical cancer with moderate to severe hemorrhagic chronic radiation proctopathy received twice-daily sucralfate enemas (20 mL of 10% suspension). By 4 months of treatment, 88.5% of these individuals experienced minimal to no hematochezia.[20] Approximately 20% of subjects experienced a rebleeding episode 5 months to 56 months after primary hemostasis, and the bleeding resolved with repeat sucralfate administration.[20] Pharmacotherapy, however, tends to have limited efficacy in patients with severe disease.[21]

An alternative treatment of severe cases is topical formalin. Formalin is a potent therapy for rectal bleeding with efficacy rates of 80% to 100%.[16] This treatment works by inducing a chemical burn.[16] During proctoscopy, 4% or buffered 10% formalin may be administered in a targeted fashion with gauze or a cotton swab, or 20 mL to 100 mL of 3.6% to 4% formalin may be applied to the affected areas.[16] After formalin application, thorough irrigation with saline to rinse away the formalin is recommended.[16] Unfortunately, formalin therapy is associated with multiple adverse effects, including perianal inflammation and discomfort, infections, delayed strictures, rectovaginal fistula formation, and necrosis, among others.[16] In addition, therapeutic results may last for only a few months.[19]

One randomized controlled trial (RCT) performed at a single referral center in India examined the success of a 4% formalin dab versus a sucralfate-steroid retention enema twice daily for 7 days to 10 days in the treatment of chronic hemorrhagic radiation proctopathy[22]; female patients post–cervical cancer treatment were evenly distributed between the treatment arms.[22] On average, hematochezia occurred a year after cessation of radiation treatment.[22] Efficacy rates of formalin and sucralfate-steroid enema were 90% and 74.5%, respectively, with individuals in the formalin arm demonstrating improved mucosal appearance post–treatment on sigmoidoscopy.[22] Those who did not achieve hemostasis with their assigned treatment subsequently underwent up to 4 additional formalin dab treatments every 14 or more days with resolution of symptoms.[22] One person who initially failed in the sucralfate-steroid enema group also failed to respond after 5 formalin applications and underwent diverting colostomy.[22] There was a small number of people with recurrent bleeding in the 2 arms (3 in the formalin and 5 in the enema groups) after a mean of 2 months, and all responded to repeat formalin administration.[22] After a mean 6-month follow-up period, no major adverse events were reported in the 2 arms, but approximately one-third of patients treated with formalin experienced minimal, self-limited discomfort.[22] Patients with the most severe endoscopic disease manifesting as deep ulcers, strictures, or fistulae[22] (ie, those most at risk for complications) were not included.[22] Thus, formalin seems to be a viable therapy in an appropriate patient population.

Endoscopic Prevention of Recurrent Bleeding

Endoscopically directed therapy for hemorrhagic radiation proctopathy is available and includes APC, heater probe, and bipolar coagulation. These are all associated with satisfactory outcomes, although it is difficult to discern the superiority of one treatment over the other in the absence of prospective trials.[16,17]

APC, as previously described, has a favorable safety profile, because its application is designed to penetrate tissue layers superficially, only up to 3 mm.[16] This is of particular importance in preventing further complications of radiation proctopathy, which is already associated with an increased incidence of fistula and stricture formation.[16] For APC use in treating radiation proctopathy, recommended settings are a flow rate of 1 L/min to 1.5 L/min and power of 40 W to 50 W, which may be escalated to 60 W in more extensive disease.[21] Up to one-fifth of patients experience an adverse event related to APC, generally mild in severity, such as fever and discomfort.[17] Serious complications, such as the development of incidental rectal ulcers,[17] luminal narrowing,[17] and, extremely uncommonly, perforation can occur.[17,21] Finally, colonic explosion has been reported in the setting of poor or incomplete bowel preparation when APC is used.[21] Luckily, this is a rare occurrence and may be avoided by use of a full bowel preparation,[21] even though the target of therapy is limited to the distal colon.

Overall, APC therapy leads to successful hemostasis in radiation proctopathy.[16] APC improves hematochezia in 80% to 90% of individuals[21] but sometimes requires repeated monthly applications.[16] In 1 small study of 28 individuals with radiation-induced rectal bleeding, patients required 1 to 8 applications of APC to achieve near or complete hemostasis with improved hemoglobins.[18] Over a mean of 40 weeks, 2 of the patients experienced rebleeding and required repeated APC treatments.[18] No major adverse events occurred during this study.[18]

In another larger prospective investigation of 56 men with mild to severe hemorrhagic radiation proctopathy after prostate cancer treatment, approximately 90% experienced only minimal bleeding or had total resolution of hematochezia after an average of 2 APC treatments.[23] All treatment failures (n = 6) occurred in the cohort with severe proctopathy.[23] These individuals went on to receive formalin application with improvement or resolution of symptoms.[23] Of the 38 followed for 1 year or longer, 4 individuals, who were on aspirin or anticoagulant therapy, experienced repeat episodes of hematochezia.[23]

Furthermore, APC may be used as a salvage therapy for ongoing hematochezia despite prior use of medications[18,24] and formalin administration.[25] APC and formalin use seem to achieve comparable outcomes in the treatment of hemorrhagic radiation proctopathy, but the side-effect profile of APC tends to be more favorable.[23] In sum, APC should be selected first over other endoscopic modalities and formalin due to the extensive clinical experience with this proved treatment and overall low associated risks.[17]

For more extensive radiation proctopathy, radiofrequency ablation (RFA), cryotherapy, and formalin administration may be more suitable therapies.[16] RFA is similar to APC in its confined depth of therapy and, additionally, promotes the regeneration of squamous epithelium after treatment.[16] Both of these characteristics assist in reducing further mucosal damage, thus preventing ulcer or stricture formation.[16] In addition, recovery of the epithelial mucosa is associated with decreased recurrence of hematochezia.[19] The data overall, however, are still limited regarding use of cryoablation[19] and RFA[17] in the treatment of hemorrhagic radiation proctopathy.

Surgery

Finally, surgery is a last resort and only indicated for a minority of individuals (<10%) with radiation proctopathy.[16] The most common indications for surgery are refractory hematochezia or sequelae of chronic inflammation, that is, fistulae, perforation, and so forth.[16] Proctectomy offers definitive therapy for refractory bleeding but is associated with anastomotic leaks, perineal surgical site infections, and other adverse events in up to 80% of patients and death rates of 3% to 9%.[16] Generally, a loop ileostomy or colostomy does not have a major role in achieving hemostasis.[16]

In sum, a stepwise approach should be pursued when treating chronic hemorrhagic radiation proctopathy.[17] Medications should be used first when feasible, followed by APC for persistent bleeding.[17,19] In situations of extensive, severe, or difficult to treat proctopathy, formalin[23] may be an option as well as RFA[19] and cryoablation.[19]

Postpolypectomy Bleeding

The rate of delayed, or nonimmediate, hemorrhage after polyp removal is 0.6% to 1.2%,[26] and this risk increases to 2.6% to 9.7% after endoscopic mucosal resection

(EMR) of polyps greater than or equal to 2 cm.[27] Risk factors for delayed postpolypectomy hemorrhage include right-sided[26,28] or pedunculated lesions,[26] large colonic polyps,[26,28] and application of low wattage coagulation energy for polypectomy.[28] Administration of coagulation current at 15 W to 20 W is believed to promote dehydration of mucosal tissue and closure of severed vasculature.[29] Postponed hemorrhage may result, however, from the transmission of energy to submucosal arteries that are susceptible to bleeding as the postpolypectomy scar is formed.[29] Conversely, cutting and blended settings generally induce earlier postpolypectomy hemorrhage.[29] Most endoscopists prefer either sole coagulation or blended energy.[29]

ENDOSCOPIC PREVENTION OF PRIMARY DELAYED POSTPOLYPECTOMY BLEEDING

The benefit of placement of endoscopic clips for the treatment of postpolypectomy bleeding is well established, but its role in primary prophylaxis against delayed LGIB after colonic EMR of sessile or flat polyps is less clear[28] and warrants exploration (**Figs. 4** and **5**).

In a 2016 meta-analysis, involving 12 studies (including 4 RCTs) and more than 18,000 polypectomies, there was no benefit found in placement of prophylactic postpolypectomy clips to prevent delayed hemorrhage.[26] This study, however, did not distinguish between polypectomies carried out via standard snare polypectomy or EMR nor did it stratify for polyp size.[26] In a subgroup analysis examining polyps greater than 2 cm in size, there was a nonstatistically significant trend in favor of a reduction in delayed hemorrhage with clipping.[26] The included studies, however, were heterogeneous in their method of polypectomy and their use of prophylactic clipping,[26] potentially limiting the ability to discern a relationship between polyp size, postpolypectomy clipping, and bleeding.

The data for prophylactic endoscopic clipping may be more favorable for EMR of large, sessile, or flat polyps. In a retrospective investigation performed at a high-volume tertiary-care center, study investigators examined rates of delayed LGIB after EMR with low-wattage coagulation current of sessile or flat polyps greater than or equal to 2 cm.[30] Approximately half of the 524 treated polyps underwent full (n = 225) or partial (n = 52) prophylactic clipping and the remainder (n = 247) were not clipped.[30] The incidence of nonimmediate bleeding was approximately 6% overall, with 24 bleeding episodes occurring in those polyps not clipped, 3 in those partially clipped, and 4 in those fully clipped.[30] The average polyp size was 3.1 cm.[30] Also, all patients without a compelling indication to be on aspirin (ie, known cardiovascular disease, including coronary artery disease, cerebrovascular accident, or transient ischemic attack) were instructed to discontinue aspirin 2 weeks prior to the procedure.[30]

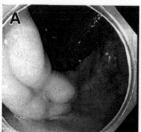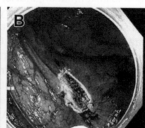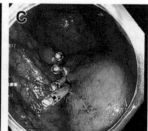

Fig. 4. (*A*) A 1-cm sessile cecal polyp (Paris class 0-IIb) removed via EMR. (*B*) Post-EMR site with evidence of mucosal defect without active bleeding. (*C*) Prophylactic postpolypectomy clips placed to decrease the risk of delayed bleeding.

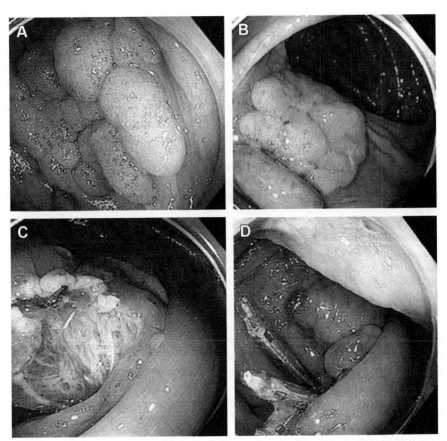

Fig. 5. (*A, B*) A 2-cm laterally spreading ascending colon tumor (Paris class 0-IIa) removed completely via piecemeal EMR. (*C, D*) Visible postpolypectomy mucosal defect prophylactically clipped to prevent delayed hemorrhage.

Further support for prophylactic clipping comes from the Spanish EMR Group, including gastroenterologists at 23 facilities in Spain, who analyzed the risk of postpolypectomy bleeding after EMR of polyps greater than or equal to 2 cm in size (n = 1255 lesions).[27] Similarly to the previous study, the average polyp was 3.1 cm in size.[27] In 67% of polypectomies, the mixture used for injection to achieve a submucosal lift included adrenaline at a concentration of 1:10,000.[27] In addition, in 6.7% of these polypectomies, APC was used solely for coagulation.[27] The incidence of immediate post-EMR bleed was 5.3%.[27] The overall incidence of delayed hemorrhage (occurring ≤15 days after completion of the procedure) was 3.7%, specifically having an impact in 1.4% in the fully clipped, 5.9% in the partially clipped, and 3.9% in the nonclipped groups.[27] Failure to fully clip the defect was associated with an odds ratio of 3.6 for post-EMR delayed hemorrhage.[27] On univariate analysis, there was no statistically significant association between either submucosal administration of adrenaline or application of APC and delayed post-EMR bleeding.[27] These findings are in agreement with the general literature, in which there seems to be little benefit to using either of these techniques as prophylactic measures against delayed postpolypectomy hemorrhage.[27]

Contrary to these findings, in an RCT performed by Shioji and colleagues,[31] the investigators discovered no utility in the placement of prophylactic clips in preventing delayed post-EMR hemorrhage. In this study, approximately one-third of the 413 to-tal EMRs (performed with blended current) were of pedunculated or semipeduncu-lated lesions.[31] Subjects were taken off antiplatelet agents and anticoagulants as medically feasible 7 days prior to the procedure and reinitiated the day after the co-lonoscopy.[31] Polyps exceeding 3 cm that were removed via piecemeal EMR were omitted from this trial because these lesions are often associated with residual polyp.[31] Presumably, the investigators were concerned that endoscopic clipping would interfere with adenoma surveillance or treatment on follow-up colonoscopy. There were only 4 instances of nonimmediate postpolypectomy hemorrhage, split evenly between the 2 respective arms (clip vs no clip).[31] As even the study investi-gators point out, however, the average polyp size was comparatively small (only 7.8 mm), which generally confers a decreased risk of delayed bleeding.[31] Thus, the study may not have been in the best position to detect a true benefit for preemp-tive clipping.[31]

Although the use of prophylactic postpolypectomy clipping can still be debated, one reasonable approach is to place endoscopic clips for significant mucosal defects, particularly in the right colon and in those individuals resuming anticoagulation or nonaspirin antiplatelet agents postprocedure.[30]

In addition, an important consideration is whether the placement of prophylactic post-polypectomy clips has an impact on the detection of persistent adenoma or new adeno-matous growth at EMR sites.[32] A prospective Australian colonic EMR study sought to determine whether stepwise use of high definition white light and narrow band imaging on the first follow-up colonoscopy enhances identification of adenomatous tissue post-EMR of laterally spreading polyps 2 cm or greater in size.[32] In 28 of 183 resected polyps, clips were placed as prophylaxis against or for therapeutic control of GIB or for closure of a mucosal defect.[32] Post-EMR scar clip artifact (ESCA) developed in approximately half of these patients.[32] ESCA delineates raised normal colonic mucosa, including gran-ulation tissue, at the post-EMR scar site secondary to clip deployment.[33]

Using standard white light endoscopy in conjunction with narrow band imaging, ESCA was identified in 96.4% of patients (in 1 case ESCA was mistaken for an ade-noma).[32] In approximately one-fifth of the subjects with ESCA, adenoma was found on biopsy of the post-EMR scar.[32] Findings from this study suggest that ESCA may be accurately distinguished with this dual imaging technique and does not inhibit the identification of adenomatous tissue at post-EMR sites.[32]

These results were corroborated in a large retrospective analysis performed by Ponugoti and Rex[28] over a 10-year period. The study investigators examined the prevalence of residual clips with or without persistent polypoid tissue at the point of clip insertion during surveillance colonoscopy after EMR of large polyps ($\geq$2 cm).[28] An average of 4 clips were placed at 479 postpolypectomy sites specifically to avoid iatrogenic LGIB.[28] Care was taken not to deploy clips at the exact locations where APC had been used to destroy residual polyp postsnaring, because these are known areas for retained or recurrent adenoma.[28] A clip adherence rate of approximately 5% was demonstrated at the initial surveillance endoscopy (performed an average 6 months later), and no residual or recurrent polyp (serrated or tubular adenoma) was diagnosed endoscopically or histologically at the insertion points of these clips.[28] In the few instances where residual adenoma was detected with concurrent clips in place, the endoscopist was able to eradicate the remaining polyp with stan-dard techniques and leave the clip in situ.[28] Thus, in experienced hands, prophylac-tic endoscopic clipping to protect against delayed LGIB does not seem to be associated with significant complications, although increased costs and time must be taken into account.

ALTERNATIVE THERAPIES IN THE MANAGEMENT OF LOWER GASTROINTESTINAL BLEEDING

Mesenteric Angiography

In the event that endoscopic therapeutic modalities fail to achieve hemostasis in LGIB or cannot be pursued, angiography may be considered.[3,4] Active hemorrhage must take place at greater than 0.5 mL/min for angiography to localize a bleeding site.[1] CTA is more sensitive than transcatheter angiography, identifying bleeding at rates of 0.3 mL/min[34] and may be used if noninvasive imaging is required before angiography.[2] Angiography with transcatheter superselective embolization achieves cessation of LGIB (including small bowel sources) in 63% to 96% of patients, but recurrent hemorrhage occurs in 11% to 50% of cases.[34] The percentage of repeat bleeding after embolization is likely lower when the analysis is limited to colonic pathologies given the richer and more redundant vascularization of the small intestine.[34] For example, in 1 systematic review, the incidence of rebleeding from diverticulosis was just 15%.[35] Transcatheter embolization of the culprit vessel may result in colonic necrosis in up to one-fifth of treated patients,[1] but generally, serious ischemic events occur in less than or equal to 3% of individuals.[34] Alternatively, transcatheter instillation of vasopressin has a success rate of 90%.[1] This method is associated, however, with an elevated risk of recurrent bleeding[1]; in all-comers, the post–vasopressin bleeding rate is 22% to 71%.[12]

Surgery

Surgery for the management of LGI hemorrhage may result in adverse events in up to 60% of individuals and death in 10%.[4] Given the high associated morbidity and mortality, surgery generally should be reserved for cases refractory to either endoscopic or radiographic therapeutic interventions.[2] It is vital to identify accurately the level of the bleeding in advance to allow for a targeted resection that is effective in achieving hemostasis.[2] Rebleeding rates, however, remain high. For instance, the postsurgical rebleeding incidence for angioectasia is 5% to 30%.[13]

In 1 retrospective series examining 104 subjects admitted to a surgical service in Israel for diverticular bleeding from 1990 to 2011, approximately 10% of patients proceeded to partial or subtotal colectomy for repeat hemorrhage.[36] The incidence of recurrent diverticular hemorrhage after surgery varies by the urgency of the operation and the type of surgery performed.[37] Repeat bleeding episodes range from 0% to 14% in elective partial colectomies for an identified hemorrhage to 42% to 63% in an emergent blind segmental resection for obscure bleeding.[37] For an emergency total colectomy for unstable, unidentified bleeding, the incidence of recurrent hemorrhage is 0% to 10%, with death rates approaching 33%.[37]

Management of Antithrombotic Agents

Preventive strategies for recurrent LGIB often involve a close examination of a patient's medication list. NSAIDs have been implicated in contributing to primary and repeat LGI hemorrhage.[38] In general, NSAIDs should be discontinued if possible after an episode of LGI hemorrhage, especially for diverticular bleeding or occult or overt blood loss due to angioectasia, given their high incidence of recurrent hemorrhage.[2]

Individuals with a history of LGIB, as opposed to UGIB, on concurrent antiplatelet therapy may be more susceptible to recurrent hemorrhage.[2] This may be in part due to the relative dearth of effective secondary prevention strategies, such as Helicobacter pylori eradication and proton pump inhibitors, and the intrinsic high rebleeding incidence associated with diverticular bleeding and bleeding from angioectasia.[2] In individuals with an acute or prior presentation of LGIB and without a compelling indication for aspirin use, such as cardiovascular or cerebrovascular disease, or an elevated risk for these conditions, aspirin should be stopped.[2]

The management of other antiplatelet agents and anticoagulants is not straightforward and mandates individual judgment regarding possibility of recurrent bleed versus adverse cardiovascular event.[2] For instance, dual antiplatelet therapy is essentially a must for individuals in the 1-month window after placement of a cardiac stent due to the increased mortality and morbidity seen on aspirin alone.[2] Consequently, a discussion with a patient's other specialists is required for these more complex agents.[2] Ideally, if these medications are held and are still required, they should be restarted as soon as possible.[2] The specific timing is contingent on degree of satisfaction with primary endoscopic hemostasis, disease-specific bleed risk, and thromboembolic risk.[2]

REFERENCES

1. Alexander J. Nonvariceal gastrointestinal tract bleeding. In: Hauser SC, editor. Mayo clinic gastroenterology and hepatology board review. 5th edition. New York: Oxford University Press; 2015. p. 123–4.
2. Strate LL, Gralnek IM. Management of patients with acute lower gastrointestinal bleeding. Am J Gastroenterol 2016;111(4):459–74.
3. Ríos R, Montoya M, Rodríguez J, et al. Severe acute lower gastrointestinal bleeding: risk factors for morbidity and mortality. Langenbecks Arch Surg 2007;392:165–71.
4. Strate LL, Naumann CR. The role of colonoscopy and radiologic procedures in the management of acute lower intestinal bleeding. Clin Gastroenterol Hepatol 2010;8:333–43.
5. Anthony T, Penta P, Todd RD, et al. Rebleeding and survival after acute lower gastrointestinal bleeding. Am J Surg 2004;188(5):485–90.
6. Yamada A, Niikura R, Yoshida S, et al. Endoscopic management of colonic diverticular bleeding. Dig Endosc 2015;27:721–6.
7. Ishii N, Setoyama T, Deshpande G, et al. Endoscopic band ligation for colonic diverticular hemorrhage. Gastrointest Endosc 2012;75(2):382–7.
8. Ishii N, Hirata N, Omata F, et al. Location in the ascending colon is a predictor of refractory colonic diverticular hemorrhage after endoscopic clipping. Gastrointest Endosc 2012;76:1175–81.
9. Aytac E, Stocchi L, Gorgun E, et al. Risk of recurrence and long-term outcomes after colonic diverticular bleeding. Int J Colorectal Dis 2014;29:373–8.
10. Sami SS, Al-Araji SA, Ragunath K. Review article: gastrointestinal angiodysplasia - pathogenesis, diagnosis and management. Aliment Pharmacol Ther 2014;39(1): 15–34.
11. Swanson E, Mahgoub A, MacDonald R, et al. Medical and endoscopic therapies for angiodysplasia and gastric antral vascular ectasia: a systematic review. Clin Gastroenterol Hepatol 2014;12(4):571–82.
12. Sharma R, Gorbien MJ. Angiodysplasia and lower gastrointestinal tract bleeding in elderly patients. Arch Intern Med 1995;155:807–11.
13. Fogel R, Valdivia EA. Bleeding angiodysplasia of the colon. Curr Treat Options Cardiovasc Med 2002;5(3):225–30.
14. Saperas E, Videla S, Dot J, et al. Risk factors for recurrence of acute gastrointestinal bleeding from angiodysplasia. Eur J Gastroenterol Hepatol 2009;21:1333–9.
15. Richter JM, Christensen MR, Colditz GA, et al. Angiodysplasia - natural history and efficacy of therapeutic interventions. Dig Dis Sci 1989;34(10):1542–6.

16. Sarin A, Safar B. Management of radiation proctitis. Gastroenterol Clin North Am 2013;42(4):913–25.
17. Weiner JP, Wong AT, Schwartz D, et al. Endoscopic and non-endoscopic approaches for the management of radiation-induced rectal bleeding. World J Gastroenterol 2016;22(31):6972–86.
18. Silva R, Correia AJ, Dias LM, et al. Argon plasma coagulation therapy for hemorrhagic radiation proctosigmoiditis. Gastrointest Endosc 1999;50(2):221–4.
19. Rustagi T, Mashimo H. Endoscopic management of chronic radiation proctitis. World J Gastroenterol 2011;17(41):4554–62.
20. Kochhar R, Sriram PVJ, Sharma SC, et al. Natural history of late radiation proctosigmoiditis treated with topical sucralfate suspension. Dig Dis Sci 1999;44(5):973–8.
21. Postgate A, Saunders B, Tjandra J, et al. Argon plasma coagulation in chronic radiation proctitis. Endoscopy 2007;39:361–5.
22. Ramakrishnaiah VPN, Javali TD, Dharanipragada K, et al. Formalin dab, the effective way of treating hemorrhagic radiation proctitis: a randomized trial from a tertiary care hospital in South India. Colorectal Dis 2012;14(7):876–82.
23. Karamanolis G, Triantafyllou K, Tsiamoulos Z, et al. Argon plasma coagulation has a long-lasting therapeutic effect in patients with chronic radiation proctitis. Endoscopy 2009;41:529–31.
24. Taieb S, Rolachon A, Cenni JC, et al. Effective use of argon plasma coagulation in the treatment of severe radiation proctitis. Dis Colon Rectum 2001;44(12):1766–71.
25. Tjandra JJ, Sengupta S. Argon plasma coagulation is an effective treatment for refractory hemorrhagic radiation proctitis. Dis Colon Rectum 2001;44(12):1759–65.
26. Boumitri C, Fazia MA, Ashraf I, et al. Prophylactic clipping and post-polypectomy bleeding: a meta-analysis and systematic review. Ann Gastroenterol 2016;29(4):502–8.
27. Albéniz E, Fraile M, Ibáñez B, et al. A scoring system to determine risk of delayed bleeding after endoscopic mucosal resection of large colorectal lesions. Clin Gastroenterol Hepatol 2016;14(8):1140–7.
28. Ponugoti PL, Rex DK. Clip retention rates and rates of residual polyp at the base of retained clips on colorectal EMR sites. Gastrointest Endosc 2017;85(3):530–4.
29. Farin G, Grund KE. Principles of electrosurgery, laser, and argon plasma coagulation with particular regard to colonoscopy [Chapter 26]. In: Waye JD, Rex DK, Williams CB, editors. Colonoscopy. principles and practice. 2nd edition. Hoboken (NJ): Wiley-Blackwell; 2009. p. 328–45.
30. Liaquat H, John E, Rex D. Prophylactic clip closure reduced the risk of delayed post-polypectomy hemorrhage: experience in 277 clipped large sessile or flat colorectal lesions and 247 control lesions. Gastrointest Endosc 2013;77(3):401–7.
31. Shioji K, Suzuki Y, Kobayashi M, et al. Prophylactic clip application does not decrease delayed bleeding after colonoscopic polypectomy. Gastrointest Endosc 2003;57(6):691–4.
32. Desomer L, Tutticci N, Tate DH, et al. A standardized imaging protocol is accurate in detecting recurrence after EMR. Gastrointest Endosc 2017;85(3):518–26.
33. Pellisé M, Desomer L, Burgess NG, et al. The influence of clips on scars after EMR: clip artifact. Gastrointest Endosc 2016;83(3):608–16.
34. Darcy MD, Cash BD, Feig BW, et al. Radiologic management of lower gastrointestinal tract bleeding. In: American College of Radiology ACR Appropriateness Criteria. 2006. Available at: https://acsearch.acr.org/docs/69457/Narrative/. Accessed October 30, 2017.

35. Khanna A, Ognibene SJ, Koniaris LG. Embolization as first-line therapy for diverticulosis-related massive lower gastrointestinal bleeding: evidence from a meta-analysis. J Gastrointest Surg 2005;9(3):343–52.
36. Gilshtein H, Kluger Y, Khoury A, et al. Massive and recurrent diverticular hemorrhage, risk factors and treatment. Int J Surg 2016;33:136–9.
37. Maykel JA, Opelka FG. Colonic diverticulosis and diverticular hemorrhage. Clin Colon Rectal Surg 2004;17(3):195–204.
38. Aoki T, Nagata N, Niikura R, et al. Recurrence and mortality among patients hospitalized for acute lower gastrointestinal bleeding. Clin Gastroenterol Hepatol 2015;13:488–94.

Moving?

Make sure your subscription moves with you!

To notify us of your new address, find your **Clinics Account Number** (located on your mailing label above your name), and contact customer service at:

Email: journalscustomerservice-usa@elsevier.com

800-654-2452 (subscribers in the U.S. & Canada)
314-447-8871 (subscribers outside of the U.S. & Canada)

Fax number: 314-447-8029

Elsevier Health Sciences Division
Subscription Customer Service
3251 Riverport Lane
Maryland Heights, MO 63043

*To ensure uninterrupted delivery of your subscription, please notify us at least 4 weeks in advance of move.